MAKING EATING RIGHT EASY

An Easy to Read Guide for those with Metabolic Syndrome:
The Condition of Having Diabetes and Hypertension

Cynthia Bland

Vabella Publishing
P.O. Box 1052
Carrollton, Georgia 30112

©Copyright 2015 by Cynthia Bland

All rights reserved. No part of the book may be reproduced or utilized in any form or by any means without permission in writing from the author. All requests should be addressed to the publisher.

Cover design by Tina Gillard.

Manufactured in the United States of America

13-digit ISBN 978-1-938230-96-7

Library of Congress Control Number 2015906551

10 9 8 7 6 5 4 3 2 1

Dedications

To my children, grandchildren and great-grandchildren who have Metabolic Syndrome or are genetically prone to "suffering" from it.

To my sisters and their children and grandchildren who might "suffer" the same fate because of genetics.

To the Community of Unhealthy Americans who want to live a long life but truly have no idea of how to provide a healthy lifestyle for themselves and their families.

Contents

Acknowledgments vii

Foreword ix

Introduction: My Story xvi

Let's Get Started 1

    Understanding Commonly Used Terminology 5

    Understanding Nutrition Labels 10

    Essential Nutrients and the
        Foods That Provide Them 16

    Deadly Food Ingredients in the Food You Buy -
        Know Them! AVOID Them! 25

    Substitutions for Deadly Food Products 28

Now Let's Shop 30

Now Let's Cook 33

Recipe Section

    Healthy Entrees 44

    Healthy Vegetable and Grain Sides 77

    Sandwiches and Quick Fixes 99

    Healthy Dips, Dressings and Sauces 105

    Healthy Snacks 111

    Delicious and Healthy Desserts 113

Let's Drink and Be Merry 134

Doing What We Love to Hate 136

My Alpha ... My Beginning 139

Learn It! Think It! Live It!
    Success is Around the Corner 140

Epilogue – Learn It! Think It! Live It!
    Success is Around the Corner 143

Works Cited 145

Acknowledgements

I thank my sister, Honora Taylor, for not only reading my guide, but for her editing and wonderful commentary which appears on the back cover. She has been unwavering in her encouragement to complete and publish this work. I had put in on the back burner warming, probably forever, until she expressed how many people she'd talked to about this work and how interested they were in getting a copy … immediately!

I thank my daughter, Payge Thomas, for not only reading my guide, but the hard work she did in editing the whole thing. Most encouraging was her comment, "I like it. There are several recipes that I'm going to prepare, especially the candy." This coming from someone who suffers from Metabolic Syndrome" and utterly resistant to anything that looks like a "diet." She makes me happy that I finished it and hopeful that it will be helpful to thousands, maybe millions.

My many thanks to Harlem Howard, my daughter, for marketing this guide before its completion because she believes in my desire to make this world healthy. Her encouragement and excitement fueled my drive to complete this guide and to believe it would be published.

Thank you to my son, Warren Maurice Nolan, for his constant and constructive advice. He makes sure that I always know what legalities are to be addressed. He insists that I be the business woman I have to be, even though he has the "business head." He keeps my head out of the clouds and makes me stand firm on the reality of the workings of the world.

Thank you to my daughter, Timi Nolan-Hudson, who takes care of my technology. She makes me check my emails, makes me send them and if I ever become overwhelmed in this cyber world, she makes it all "real" for me.

I thank Jerome Henson for taking on the task of formatting this guide. He never spoke of any payment but immediately took on this formidable task.

I thank Tina Gillard who, also, without any talk of payment took on the task of graphic artist, designing my covers and enhancing the photos of the prepared food products in the recipe section of the guide.

Most importantly, I thank God for the wisdom, strength and faith to tackle this endeavor with great joy. I thank Him for sending His angels to gather around me. Hallelujah!

Foreword

Metabolic Syndrome and Obesity Do Not Have to Be Killers

I am a 73 year old African-American woman who was diagnosed with diabetes and borderline hypertension at the age of 62. I wasn't surprised with the diagnosis of diabetes but hypertension was a scary thing. I expected to have to deal with diabetes because it didn't skip a generation in our family. Having been reared with and then ultimately having to care for my brother who was a juvenile diabetic, not expected to live past 30 years of age, I was certain that I'd live to a ripe old age, after all, he'd lived to 56 and was just beginning to experience complications. I measured how long I'd be able to live and computed my longevity to be no less than 92. They say that women live as long as their mothers, so I knew 91 years, at least, would be the time for me to go and meet my Father face-to-face.

On the issue of hypertension, my father died at 58 years of age due to complications of hypertension. He'd had a couple of strokes and then ultimately died of kidney failure. Too young to die, but his lifestyle made understanding his early demise as a reasonable event.

My father ate all of the wrong foods and even though my mom prepared him the best low-fat and saltless meals, he couldn't let his favorite "tastes" go. I didn't know enough about hypertension or diabetes to aid him or my brother. I just knew that they both had deadly diseases.

I was able to glean from the many discussions I'd heard between my mom and dad that hypertension could be corrected if salt and alcoholic beverages were used in moderation and stress were eliminated as much as possible. The question remained in my psyche, "What is moderation?"

I didn't know that diet and exercise was the only "cure." Both, my dad and brother, would have lived longer if anyone had known how the diseases "worked" and if they'd been willing to make necessary changes.

I would often ask my brother what his doctors recommended to insure a longer life. His response was always, "My doctors always tell me that I know more about diabetes than they do." They just checked his vitals, refilled his prescriptions for insulin and sent him on his way. When I began going to the same clinic as he did, expecting more answers regarding treatment, I was disappointed. The best that I was offered was an off-handed invitation to come to the nutrition classes. I accepted the menus and diets but didn't understand how to figure out the "exchanges" thing. I was in the same position as my brother – fishing in the dark, hoping to catch the big one.

For years I just took my Metformin, ate less food, continued exercising and avoided alcoholic beverages. The best thing that I had on my side was the grave fear of death that had haunted me all of my life. My doctor required that I visited the office every 3 months to check my vitals and get my A1C checked. My A1C started out at about 8 and slowly went down. My doctor's only advice, "I want your A1C at 7."

Again, I didn't understand what A1C was, what its importance was, and how to get it down. Because there was no help forthcoming, I decided to get the information on my own. I began researching the "cure." I adjusted and readjusted the foods that I prepared and ate. It was time consuming, at times extremely frustrating and painful but I got it. It took me a total of 6 years to get my disease under control but finally, I owned it; it no longer owned me.

In the interim of the 6 years, my brother had many stays in the cardiac unit of the hospital suffering from complications. No "cure." No direct information. They would stabilize him, he'd come home and we'd ride the same roller coaster ride until the next time he had an insulin reaction and/or seizures that would deem him unresponsive and needing another few days stay to get regulated. Finally, his number came up.

We'd moved into a new home where he insisted on helping move boxes. I saw him struggling with a box and told him to stop and sit down. He took it up the 5 steps and then went to his room to lie down for 20 minutes before dinner. A bit later, I called him to dinner. He did not respond, so I went to his new room expecting him to be asleep. He was. He was enjoying his final earthly sleep. His heart had given out.

I was committed to never having to go through what he went through. I knew there had to be answers somewhere to assist me in my quest to be "cured." One doctor told me there was no cure. He said that I'd be diabetic all of my life, dependent on medications and a diabetic diet.

I started looking for definitions of diabetic concern: carbohydrates, calories, sugar, A1C; and then hypertension terminology: cholesterol, lipids, triglycerides HDL, LDL; finally, I researched all of the terms used to explain my kidney function: creatine, protein, albumin. I sought to understand what the doctor was looking for in my quarterly vital levels.

The answers I found could have scared me and put me in a state of denial which would lead to an untimely death or could be used to help me pursue and sustain a healthy lifestyle. I didn't have to have insulin reactions. I didn't have to suffer seizures. I didn't have to endure amputation of my lower limbs. I didn't have to endure dialysis, be disabled or die. I found that all I had to do was eat right, maintain a healthy weight and exercise regularly.

I vowed to make sure that my children would not have to stop living their lives to take care of me because I didn't know how to live a healthy life. Diabetes nor hypertension was going to take me out!

The 2012 diabetic community as illustrated in the National Diabetes Statistics Report, 6/10/2014, shows the following:
- 9.3% (29.1million) of the total population were diabetic
- Prevalence of seniors age 65 and up – 25.9 or 11.8 million, diagnosed and undiagnosed
- Prediabetic – 86 million age 20 and up
- 7.6% diabetics are Caucasians
- 9% diabetics are Asian American
- 12.8% diabetics are Hispanic
- 13.2% diabetics are African Americans
- 15.9% diabetics are American Indians/Alaskan natives
- Diabetics, age 20 and up account for 282,000 emergency room visits
- 71% of diabetics, age 18 and up, have hypertension
- 65% of diabetics, age 18 and up, have high Lower Density Lipid (LDL) readings or used cholesterol lowering medication
- Diabetics, age 20 and up, suffer 1.8 times more heart attacks than non-diabetics.
- Diabetics account for 44% of all newly diagnosed kidney failure (2011)
- Diabetics, age 20 and up, suffer strokes 1.5 times high than non-diabetics
- Diabetics, age 20 and up, account for 73,000 non-traumatic lower limb amputations
- Diagnosed diabetics account for $245 billion of total medical care (3-6-2013)
- Diabetics spend $176 billion for direct medical costs
- Diabetics account for $69 billion in lost wages due to reduced productivity directly related to complications of diabetes: dialysis, blindness, loss of limbs, and heart disease (American Diabetes Association, 2014)

The questions that you have to ask yourself are, "Where am I in these statistics? What can I do, myself, to make a difference in the way I live out my life?"

The warnings of impending disability and complications of these diseases (heart attacks, strokes, kidney disease and the loss of limbs) only serve to discourage rather than inspire patients to believe that only a commitment to a healthy existence is needed to change the course of these diseases. It is true that there is no cure for these diseases, but remission can be achieved with a simple lifestyle change.

Why live with the threat of complications due to diabetes and hypertension when the solution to controlling them is to simply eat right and exercise just 20 minutes a day. The best "cure" for these diseases is education coupled with a healthy dose of self-control.

My medical provider finally referred me to an endocrinologist, a specialist of the endocrine system, which includes the pancreas, the organ that was not functioning properly which causes diabetes. He listened to me express my fears and then gave me some goals to reach and some answers to my previously unanswered questions. I continued my research. I read every pamphlet that I saw in doctors' offices and then researched everything that the pamphlets and articles didn't explain to my satisfaction. Diabetes and hypertension began to take on a new face. They did not look like the grim reaper anymore; they began to look like the giant did to David – something I could beat!

When my endocrinologist exclaimed, "I want to clone you!" I was excited beyond belief. My A1C was 5.9, my waistline measured ½ of my height, my vitals levels were all in the "healthy" range. I had succeeded by changing my diet and by exercising regularly. He so motivated me that I made my next goal to be med-free! It took another year, but it happened! I have been med free for 5 months! My medical provider told me, "You are not cured; there is no cure, but you are in remission." Fine thing! Not as encouraging as my endocrinologist, but he did admit that I could be med free. I am only taking my low dose aspirin and 2.5 mg. of Lisinopril which I take to protect my kidneys, NOT for hypertension. My blood pressure stays in the normal range!

Now I know that anyone who wants to overcome diabetes and/or hypertension and obesity can, without suffering.

This easy to read and understand pocket-sized guide was born out of the passion I have of living a long healthy, active life. I have, carved in stone, another 18 years to spend on this earth and to make a difference while doing so. The difference I can make is to share my "cure" with you, the reader and user of this guide.

There are many publications that address the dietary needs of diabetics. The recipes in these publications address the carbohydrate level successfully, but the fat levels are usually higher than I would ever want to consume. At the end of each recipe, the usual nutritional count is provided, however, is not helpful unless the patient understands how to determine the impact of the meal on their condition. The serving size on the nutritional guide does not specify the recommended serving size for those who suffer from diabetes and/or hypertension and obesity. Additionally, the recipes are often designed in the test kitchens of major food manufacturers and thus suggest the use of prepared and/or processed foods that contain harmful chemicals and other dangerous additives.

The seemingly unending roller coaster that people with these diseases are condemned to ride can be a smooth and steady uphill climb to a comfortable plateau of balanced healthy blood sugar levels and safe blood pressure readings if the "owners" of these diseases take the reins and run the race with an "I can do it!" attitude.

This pocket-sized guide contains information that food manufacturers don't want the consumers of their products to know about. The government issued mandates regulating the packaging, nutrition and ingredient labeling that food manufacturers must adhere to, but too many consumers do not understand the scientific terminology or the mathematical operations that have to be implemented for them to be useful. This guide makes the computation of total carbs, appropriate serving sizes, and good vs. bad fat content simple. It also helps with meal planning, in that it includes healthy substitutions that replace animal fats and limit the use of natural and artificial sweeteners. Finally, this guide offers a thorough list of vitamins and minerals that are found in food products and that the body needs to maintain healthy organ function.

My Story

I began my quest for a healthy lifestyle when, nine years ago, my doctor told me that I was diabetic and borderline hypertensive. Me! High blood pressure??? How in the world did I get myself into this mess? Diabetes runs in our family like our red hair so I felt it was a more normal occurrence, but hypertensive? How unfair.

I left the doctor's office armed with my prescription for Metformin to do something. You're right – I had no idea of what I was supposed to do or what the medicine was supposed to do. I just knew I had to do something and it had to do something. The only question I could ponder was, "Was the medicine going to cure me of diabetes?"

My mind whirled. What could I do to prevent going over the line and become full-fledged hypertensive? What could I do to cure my diabetes? I didn't think about controlling either; I wanted them to go away. I suppose my thoughts were more in line with denial than in the need to change my lifestyle. After all, I didn't do anything at all to fall victim to these dreadful diseases.

My doctor informed me that there was no cure for diabetes; I didn't know that. I had no idea that it was a progressive disease. I did know that I could live with the disease because there was no prognosis of "terminal." I walked away thinking that I could not stop the disease from affecting my whole physical being. My overall well-being was in jeopardy. I walked away feeling depressed and defeated.

Having lived with my brother, who was afflicted with juvenile diabetes at the age of nine, I came to understand that low blood sugar was not good, nor was high blood sugar, but I had no idea of what consequence vacillating between the two could be. I didn't realize that there had to be a balance and that healthy blood sugar levels had to be between 90 and 120. I didn't realize that going into the 190 – 200 range meant that my blood would be thicker than it should be in the lower, healthy range. I didn't know what spiking was and how it affected the whole body. I wasn't taught that spiking meant that the food that my brother had eaten would raise his blood sugar into the 200s, then upon discovering how high his blood sugar was, computing how much insulin he needed by using a sliding scale that his diabetic nurse taught me to use would lower it requiring that he eat again. What a roller coaster ride! I was learning step-by-step how this disease behaved. I learned a little, but there was no cohesion in my instruction. I was always, whether it was his or my health issue, learning from event to event. There were classes on diet and nutrition that we could have attended, but there didn't seem to be a great need for us to attend. The classes were announced in bulletins, pamphlets and diabetic guides, but the sense of urgency was not in them. It all seemed off-handed advice, more like invitations. I didn't understand the need for me to change my whole lifestyle. I felt that I could be a healthy diabetic all by myself. Just walk away from sweet things.

What I didn't know was more important than what I did know. I didn't understand the conversion of carbs into the deadly "sugar." I didn't understand that fructose, the "sugar" that is in fruit and some vegetables, could be one of the deadly "sugars" that I had to avoid. Potatoes are not sweet, but carbs galore! Deadly "sugar." My brother would often look at my dinner plate and with that smile that would creep over his face turning him from a mature man into a little imp, would say, "That is not the plate of a diabetic." I think he got great joy from being able to admonish me. The table had turned and now he could teach me how hard being a diabetic could be. Weighing food, vegetables for snacks, counting exchanges. I got the "counting exchanges," but once again, diabetic terminology wasn't what I was trying to master. I just wanted to know how to fix my plate so that it wasn't a horror movie. I didn't want to see the grim reaper's face smiling at me out of the mashed potatoes and gravy.

I knew that it was a fact that while doctors are knowledgeable professionals on whom we depend for our general well-being, most of them do not know a lot about diabetes. The specialists that do know a lot about diabetes are endocrinologists, doctors who specialize in the workings of the endocrine system. They know how our glands work. They know the symptoms of different gland malfunction and what symptoms indicate trouble; but because more research must be done to uncover the mysteries of the pancreas' function, they can only help us to control our levels by running our blood tests and interpreting the results.

So much of this disease's behavior had to be learned by trial and error. I had to become more familiar with the "workings" of my body to learn to treat my diabetes with respect. I had to learn to fear diabetes because it could become the thing that would take me down a road that I dreaded having to tread. I accepted the fact that I was on the road, then I focused on navigating it to a positive destination.

I discovered that a lot of the recipes created especially for diabetics did not work for me, and most, while dealing with cutting carbs and sugar, they did not address metabolic syndrome. Too much fat was all that I could see. What a dilemma! I realized that I would have to do my own research and attack diabetes as if I were fighting for my life. I was.

I started with Googling "foods that have cholesterol." Everything that I loved jumped onto to screen! Basically, for me, it meant never enjoying food again. It wasn't the worst thought ever, I was at a lifetime high weight of 174 pounds. Just 54 pounds to lose to regain my high school graduation weight. Hah! I knew about the no salt thing, but potato chips was my favorite food! Regardless of the fat and salt, chips were something that I felt I could eat if I'd just wipe the salt off and enjoy them plain or buy salsa to dip them in. Tomato products are valuable in that they have a lot of nutritional value so I decided that I could reduce the peril of eating them by relying on the antioxidants to gather up all of the fat and run it out of my body ... Wrong! Potato chips would become my once a month treat and only ten, as a serving, with the salt wiped off. Just a little salt won't kill. Like the Lord says, "All things in moderation."

Even though moderation appeared really small on my plate, my body learned to require less of everything. God created the human body to adjust to its environment and mine had to adjust to a sugar-free and fat-free one. What an awful task! The people with whom I lived still wanted to enjoy their favorite foods and I, often, had to be the one to cook them without preaching about moderation. I had to learn to at least substitute the "dangerous" foods with "safe" foods.

I had no idea that the grocery store would become my nutrition library. My daughters warned whoever had the task of taking me to the library, chiding me, "Mom is going to read every label, compute the prices, read the ingredients list, and study the nutrition labels. Then after all that, decide to cook everything from scratch!"

The more I studied the labels and then researched the additives, preservatives, artificial colors and chemicals to "preserve freshness or worse to make my food look fresh and vibrant", the more important shopping correctly became my health's salvation.

My interest in blood pressure health peaked at the revelation that I might actually need to be concerned. I looked at the American Heart Association recommendation for healthy blood pressure. The AHA listed blood pressure categories as:

- Normal – Systolic less than 120; diastolic less than 80
- Prehypertension – Systolic 120 – 139; diastolic 80-89

- High Blood Pressure (Hypertension) – Stage 1- systolic 140 to 159; diastolic 90 -99
- High Blood Pressure (Hypertension) Stage 2 – systolic 160 or higher; diastolic 100 or higher
- Hypertensive Crisis (Emergency care needed) – Systolic higher than 180 or diastolic higher than 110
(Source: Mayoclinc.org)

I found out that systolic, the top number, measures the pressure in the arteries when the heart beats (when the heart contracts – pulls in or squeezes shut).

Diastolic, the bottom number measures the pressure in the arteries between heart beats (when the heart muscle is resting between beats and refilling with blood).

Because I am a very visual learner, I immediately pictured myself holding a balloon filled with water. When I contracted/squeezed the balloon nearest the tied part "artery", the "heart" became taut. When I released the part in my hand the "blood" rushed back and the balloon resumed its normal shape (resting position). That's sorta' how it works. The part I needed to "see" was how efficiently the artery under pressure responded. While this illustration will never make it to the AHA Journal, it gave me, a lay person, a picture of how an overly-taxed heart might look. Not a pretty picture. I didn't want my arteries to be under undue pressure and my heart to enlarge due to the poor release of blood back into my arteries.

I already knew that salt was dangerous and had to go. After all, salt is what is used to preserve many food products, especially meats and since my body is flesh, it only makes sense that if I indulge in a high salt diet that I am going to dry up! The picture of my arteries drying up was scary. My grandmother had arteriosclerosis (hardening of the arteries) and since we loved her dearly we didn't mind listening to the stories that were recorded in her brain and played like a tape recorder on rewind. But she would have been devastated to know that she was suffering from senile dementia. I know that I can lessen my chances of boring my children, grands and great-grands if I take some preventive measures to KEEP MY BLOOD PRESSURE AND DIABETES UNDER CONTROL.

One thing that helped me was getting an understanding of how high blood glucose could cause those possibly fatal blood clots leading to brain strokes and heart attacks. I had to get a good picture. I finally understood that high blood glucose causes the blood to thicken, and that while drinking loads of water, red wine, taking aspirin or taking insulin would be effective in thinning the blood those remedies are not in any way considered controlling your disease.

I pictured my blood as train cars being hitched to the locomotor, the life source of the train. There is the thick blood, some thin blood, some thick blood, some thin blood and as these cars proceed down the track coursing toward their destination (your brain or heart) they meet obstacles, cholesterol (a mountain); free radicals (pollutants), narrow tunnels (arteries with accumulated plaque). Are you getting the picture? Your disease can be a train wreck in the making. My lack of control/discipline could shorten my life or worse debilitate me to the point of having to be totally dependent on others for my care. My children had lives to live and I didn't want to impede their progress through life by putting them in the untenable situation of having to be concerned about my care. I knew that my greatest fear could become my reality if I didn't, immediately, change my lifestyle. I recognized that my love for them meant that I had to be committed to remaining healthy and independent.

I'm through telling you my story. Now, the book becomes focused on you joining me in the quest of good healthy eating leading to a long, healthy, independent life.

Chapter 1

Let's Get Started

You don't have to quit eating good tasting food; you just have to acquire a different taste that spells out satisfaction. I do not promise that the recipes that I offer are like restaurant entrees or like our spreads at Thanksgiving or Christmas. None of these drip in butter, have glazes that shimmer in the light of the chandelier, are basted in the animal fat that glistens on the skin of the beast that gave his/her life for your culinary pleasure. But! These are really good and healthy! If you want to add ingredients, just Google your ideas and wow! Be amazed by the offerings of folks that like food but love life more! Don't let food be your pleasure; it can be one of the things that pleases you.

Read and study the information that precedes the recipes. These are all important facts that will help you understand why specific foods and spices are so necessary in your diet. It is all really amazing! I put this together so you don't have to do a lot of work. I put it in the simplest terms. I used common everyday vocabulary so you don't have to use a dictionary, but one thing you will want to do is Google additional varieties of the foods that do the most to aid our body's organ function.

I actually started my journey on the road to perfect health at 174 pounds and I now stay at between 120 – 123 pounds and am off medication! It works. Remember! Serving sizes do matter! They matter a lot! Remember, all things in moderation! It doesn't matter how healthily you have prepared your meals if you double up on the servings. Think about it like this. If your carbohydrates (They convert to sugar.) are right at 5grams, when you double up your portion, you're looking at 10 grams! And if each gram is multiplied by 5 points, you have 50 grams of carbohydrates (almost your daily limit) on one plate! Your blood sugar skyrockets, so you have to do the most dangerous thing around your diet – fast or remedy the high blood sugar by taking a blood thinner (extra insulin, an aspirin, loads of water, 4 ounces of dry red wine). This is called spiking! The train is chugging down the track! Unlike the Little Engine That Could, No you can't, no you can't, no you can't. A diabetic must eat three small meals and two healthy low carb and low sugar snacks per day. If you have hypertension, then your meals and snacks must be low salt and low fat, also. You have to plan your day's intake of food! Yes, this is a chore sometimes, but just think of being wheelchair bound or bedridden. All of a sudden it is a joy!

Now About That Servings Thing

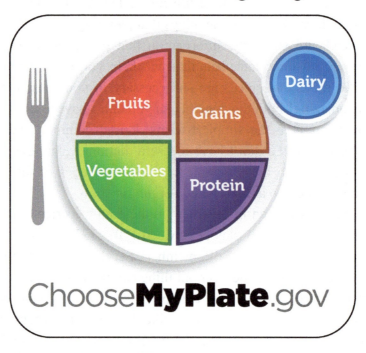

(choosemyplate.govUSDA)

Making Eating Right Easy

Study "your" plate. Your healthy plate has one thing on it that you can eat without limit. Carb and cholesterol free salads! Make a jar of the dips that you will find in the recipe section of this guide and put those on your salad. Purchase fat free mayo.

Use fat free/good fat sauces on your fish like vinaigrettes, mustard, hot sauce or tartar sauce made from scratch. You can win this battle with just a little information and a lot of self-discipline.

The meat section of your plate is one-fourth of the food allotted per meal. A three to four ounce serving is all that you are allowed daily. Meat is cholesterol. Meat is fat! You can get rid of a lot of the fat if you skin and de-fat your meat, but you will still have some fat and the cholesterol remains a problem. Try to limit your meat intake to one serving per day. NO processed meats! NO greasy sausages! Use fresh ground turkey or chicken in ALL of your recipes. NO smoked meats, including turkey! Smoked, preserved and processed meats are dangerously high in salt content and fat. The bacon, sausage and egg breakfast is called the heart attack breakfast for a reason. Become repulsed at the sight of fatty meats, including ham, on your plate. Substitute salmon croquets for fatty meats. Pan fry them in coconut or olive oil. Yummy! Grits or brown rice with a tad of butter, coconut oil or olive oil. Yummy! And healthy too!

You can have up to two servings of fish per day every day or at least three times per week; just eat the healthy fishes: mackerel, lake trout, herring, cod, tuna, anchovies, and salmon. These all are rich in Omega 3 and Omega 6; the benefits of which are great!

Remember, all things in moderation. Your stomach will shrink in a short period of time but until it does you can eat until satisfied leafy green vegetable (kale, spinach, romaine, iceburg lettuce) salads with healthy toppings, such as raisins, walnuts, ½ of a chopped boiled egg (2x a week), tomato, cucumber, green onion, mushrooms – a plate full of goodness.

A good way to estimate a serving is by using the following visual:

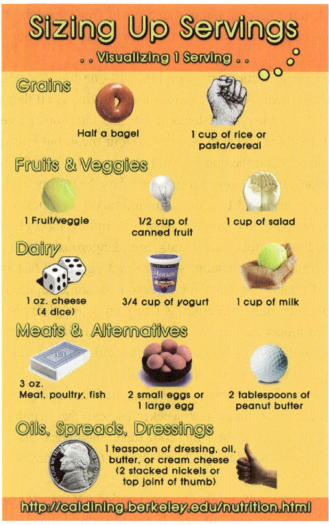

(Caldining, Berkley University n.d.)

Making Eating Right Easy
Understanding Commonly Used Terminology

The following are terms that we've heard a million times, yet have no clear definition for. I included these definitions to enhance your reading and understanding of the text of this guide.

Antioxidants- protect body from damage caused by harmful molecules which are called free radicals.
Free radicals are by-products of normal processes that take place in your body: burning of sugars for energy; release of digestive enzymes to break down food; break down of certain medicines; pollutants.
Foods that are good source of antioxidants and redirect free radicals:
Vitamin E - Nuts, seeds, olive and coconut oils, avocado, spinach, Swiss chard, almonds, asparagus.
Vitamin C – citrus fruits, broccoli.
Green Tea
B vitamins –improve unhealthy cholesterol levels
Blackstrap molasses - Reduces triglycerides in blood – dry roasted pecans, flax seed, nuts.
Damage of free radicals believed to cause macular degeneration, Alzheimer's, cancer, blood vessel disease, some arthritis-related conditions.
Atherosclerosis/ Arteriosclerosis – Hardening of the arteries. Arteries that flexibility, therefore proper function, is compromised because of a build-up of plaques (fat, cholesterol and other substances). Restricts flow of blood causing serious, possibly life-threatening conditions.
Omega 3 – Polyunsaturated fatty acid that lowers triglycerides; decreases coronary artery disease, protects against irregular heart beat and lowers blood pressure; lowers inflammation a key component in asthma.

Foods rich in Omega 3
Fish – anchovies, herring, mackerel, salmon, lake trout, sardines, tuna

Macular Degeneration = deterioration of small spot in center of retina. Causes blindness more frequently than glaucoma. Smokers beware!

Legumes (muscle carbs) - rebuild muscles after exercise; relatively no high or low glycemic (blood sugar) effect. Nuts, peas, lentils, soybeans (Combine with healthful fats and clean protein for maximum effect).

Protein – The building blocks of life. Every cell in the body contains protein. Basic structure of protein is a chain of amino acids. Protein helps your body repair cells and makes new ones. It is very important for growth and development in children, teens, and pregnant women. You do not have to eat animal products to get all the protein you need in your diet. Protein can be found in soy, beans, legumes, nut butters, and some grains: wheat germ and quinoa.

- **Enzymes** - biological molecules (proteins) that act as means to help complex reactions occur everywhere in life.
- **Casein** (slower digesting protein) - Abundant in milk; cottage cheese.
- **Clean Protein** – eggs, fish, cheese, meat

Metabolic Syndrome – A cluster of conditions: increased blood pressure, a high blood sugar level, excess body fat around the waist and abnormal cholesterol that occur together, increasing your risk of heart disease, stroke and diabetes.

Metabolism – General definition: Sum total of all of the chemical reactions in the body. To raise or speed up metabolism means, simply, to burn calories faster. Look at all of the endocrine gland functions and you can see how our thoughts, feelings, beliefs and experiences ... our lifestyle ... influence metabolism. Metabolism is defined as having two categories:

- **Catabolism** – breakdown of molecules to obtain energy.
- **Anabolism** – synthesis of all compounds needed by cells.

Endocrinologist – Medical specialist trained to diagnose and treat hormone imbalances and problems by helping to restore normal balance of hormones in the body.

Common diseases treated: diabetes and thyroid disorders; coordination of metabolism respiration, reproduction, sensory perception and movement; endocrine glands and tissue which produce hormones.

Endocrine glands
- **Pituitary** – master gland: secretes hormones that regulate function of other glands.
- **Adrenal** (atop kidneys) releases hormone (adrenaline) in response to stress; produces testosterone (identifies male characteristics) and aldosterone (kidney function).
  Iron – Reduces cough and pre-dialysis anemia and regulates metabolism.
- **Pancreas** – produces insulin to regulate carbs and fat metabolism.
- **Hypothalamus** – A part of the lower middle brain that tells the pituitary gland when to release hormones.
- **Ovaries** – The female reproductive organs that release eggs and produce sex hormones.
- **Testes** – The male reproductive glands that produce sperm and sex hormones.
- **Thymus** – A gland in the upper chest that helps develop the body's immune system early in life.
- **Thyroid** – A butterfly-shaped gland in the front of the neck that controls metabolism. It regulates blood pressure, heart rate, metabolism and body temp and how the body reacts to other hormones.

Fats/lipids: The good: They remain liquid at room temp.

Monounsaturated – improves cholesterol levels, benefit insulin levels and blood sugar control, enhances body's ability to absorb beneficial carotenoids: beta carotene, Vitamin A strengthens immune functions, skin and bones.

Polyunsaturated – plant based foods and oils improve bad cholesterol; contains Omega 3.

The bad: They are solid at room temp. When cooked greasy foods cool, the grease gets solid again.

Saturated and Trans Fats – animal fat –increases LDL cholesterol; lowers HDL cholesterol.

Diglycerides and Monoglycerides- disguised trans fat.

Triglycerides - do not dissolve in blood. Hormones release triglycerides for energy between meals. Eat more calories than you burn and triglycerides get stored in fat cells. Triglycerides respond better to dietary change than medicines. They cause hardening of arteries (atherosclerosis/arteriosclerosis).

Partially hydrogenated fat – disguised trans fat.

Soybean oil – GMO – Don't eat.

Lipoprotein – protein bonded to fatty acid.

Cholesterol/lipid – It does not dissolve in blood. It is a waxy substance made by body. If you ingest more in foods you choose, LDL increases.

Sulfites – preservatives and antioxidants – used to improve appearance. Problem only when you have food allergies or when ingested in large amts. = combination of foods containing sulfites: alcoholic beverages, peeled potato products, cheeses, seafood, canned fruit and vegs, dried fruit.

Chemicals:

Aspartame – Nutrasweet and Equal believed to be carcinogenic

High fructose Corn Syrup- GMO, increases LDL, contributes to development of diabetes and tissue damage. Don't eat.

Making Eating Right Easy

Monosodium glutamate – overexcites cells to point of damage or death, depression, disorientation, eye damage, headaches and obesity. Frustrates brain function that makes you feel full.

Food Dyes – behavioral problems in children, reduction in IQ, thyroid cancer, chromosomal damage.

Sodium sulfite – rashes, headaches, rashes.

Hydrogenated veg oils – These oils are chemically removed from vegetables and have a high concentration of Omega 6 which is bad because Omega 3 and Omega 6 have to be in balance. They are also linked to cancer.

Sodium nitrate/nitrite – Believed to cause colorectal/stomach cancer and wreaks havoc with pancreas and liver. They are found in processed, preserved or highly salted foods.

Sulfur dioxide – Causes bronchial problems, low blood pressure, destroys Vitamins B1 and E, aggravates emphysema, asthma or cardiovascular disease.

Potassium bromate – An additive used to increase volume in some breads, flour and rolls. It is believed to be carcinogenic.

Potassium sorbate, calcium sorbate, sodium sorbate are all preservatives.

Acrylamide – Believed to be Carcinogenic. They are contained in bag used for microwave popcorn.

Acrylates – in packaging of food products.

Titanium dioxide – used as whitener in paint, food coloring, sunscreens, cosmetics, pigmentation for vitamins.

BHA/BHT – Preservatives to lengthen shelf life. Effect neurological system of brain, alter behavior, and has the potential to cause cancer.

Cynthia Bland

Understanding a Nutrition Label

You will begin visiting the grocery store library. You MUST understand two things that are on every grocery item, the nutrition label and the ingredients that are in the food product. You MUST read them, study them and then make a decision to purchase the food product or cook that same food product from scratch.

It is extremely important that you understand the nutrition guide on food products. It took the health community a long time to get this information mandated for the consumer.

Nutrition Facts

Serving Size 1/2 cup (115g)
Servings Per Container About 4

Amount Per Serving

Calories 250   Calories from Fat 130

	% Daily Value*
Total Fat 14g	22%
Saturated Fat 9g	45%
Cholesterol 55mg	18%
Sodium 75mg	3%
Total Carbohydrate 26g	9%
Dietary Fiber 0g	0%
Sugars 26g	
Protein 4g	

Vitamin A 10%	Vitamin C 0%
Calcium 10%	Iron 0%

* Percent Daily Values are based on a 2,000 calorie diet.

(Nutrition Index n.d.)

Making Eating Right Easy

Let's start at the top of the Nutrition Label. The heading is Nutrition facts. Facts are proven data meaning the contents have to be scientifically computed to meet Food and Drug Administration standards.

- The first datum is **SERVING SIZE**. This guide includes a plate and chart to illustrate what your serving size is to be. Use it.
- The next datum is **SERVINGS PER CONTAINER**. Maybe you should be able to double the servings in that container. If it says a serving size is a cup, you think ½ cup per serving. Have the rest of your package serving for your snack.

Now we have the list of amounts per serving:

- **Calories** and **Calories from Fat**. This is most important information. This will determine whether or not you want to eat the product. If the calories from fat are more than 25% of the listed calories (divide the total calories by 4), put the item back on the shelf.
- **% Daily Value*** - note the *. Whenever you see an asterisk (*), LOOK DOWN! An asterisk indicates that a definition or additional detail is available – read it!

On a nutrition label the asterisk precedes this most important information. The percent daily values are based on a 2,000 calorie diet. That is a lot of food! It is for someone who is working out or super active all day, every day! There is a mathematical formula to figure out how many carbs this is, but I am committed to not making this a formidable guide and I remind you that I am not a medical professional. Therefore I am recommending that you ask your doctor how many calories or carbs he/she wants you to take in each day.

Now we're at the meat and potatoes part of the nutritional label's facts.

Total Fat – This includes saturated fat, polyunsaturated fat, unsaturated fat, monounsaturated fat and trans fat. To keep this simple, some fats are good for you; some are poison. Trans fat, partially hydrogenated and saturated fats are to be avoided like the plague.

To make this extremely complex subject really simple, I went to Mayoclinic.org. You can go there if you want to really understand all of the research done on dietary fats.

Here are the facts published by this highly-respected medical organization:

- It is wise to choose the healthier types of dietary fat and enjoy them in moderation.
- Fat is high in calories. Eat more calories than you need and you will gain weight!
- Fat and its cousin, cholesterol, play a role in cardiovascular disease and Type 2 diabetes. Bad fat, those that are solid at room temperature, are called saturated fat and trans fat. These two fats increase unhealthy LDL (low density lipoprotein) cholesterol and lower the healthy HDL (high density lipoprotein) cholesterol.
- Monounsaturated fats improve cholesterol levels and benefit insulin levels which control your blood sugar. (It is liquid at room temperature so it stays liquid at normal body temperature. Makes sense that it is not in your body getting hard and sticking to the sides of your arteries.)
- Polyunsaturated, plant-based foods and oils improve bad cholesterol; decrease the risk of heart disease and Type 2 diabetes. Polyunsaturated fat contains Omega 3, which decreases coronary artery disease, protects against irregular

Making Eating Right Easy

heartbeats and lowers blood pressure. (Again, get the picture! It is liquid at room temperature so it stays liquid at normal body temperature. It only makes sense that it is not in your body getting hard and sticking to the sides of your arteries.)
- The total fat for a person on a 2000 calorie diet is 44 – 78 grams per day. Since we are trying to lose weight and gain control of our diabetes and blood pressure, we are going to cut the calorie diet to 1000, so 22 – 39 grams of fat per day will be sufficient to remain healthy.
- Trans fat is partially hydrogenated fat which is saturated fat. If the product you are thinking about purchasing has monoglycerides or diglycerides in the ingredients section, you are purchasing a product that has trans fat. The FDA allows food manufacturers/producers to disguise trans fats as mono- or diglycerides! Look for this ingredient on every product label. If it is listed, DO NOT BUY or USE.
- Soybean oil is manmade, do not eat.
- Canola oil is a GMO – genetically modified organism. It is the least dangerous oil, but if you can, try to use only olive oil or coconut oil.
- These bad fats are found in ice cream, cakes, cookies, pie, margarine and spreads, ready-to-use frosting, coffee creamers and frozen pizza. Cook from scratch.
- Stop eating The 3 Ps: prepared, preserved and or processed foods.

When I worked at a popular department store as a stock person, I had to check products to make sure the expiration date had not been passed. What I discovered was that the shelf life for most food products was more than a year. What distressed me was the shelf life for baby food was up to four years. Think about what that means in terms of your children's health. The chemicals used. It is sinful. Any food that doesn't spoil soon after preparation or after being picked has to be dangerous. It is not natural for food products to last that long. Frozen food has a freezer life of no more than 6 months. If it is in a can, box or jar on the store shelf. Don't buy it!

Cholesterol is not fat. It is a waxy, fat-like substance that your body makes enough of to meet your needs, but excess cholesterol increases LDL. Most foods with saturated fats have cholesterol. Keep cholesterol at 0 - < 5 (less than 5) milligrams per serving.
- You want to keep your cholesterol at less than 200 milligrams per day, so consume food products that contain monounsaturated or polyunsaturated fats instead of fatty foods. Remember that we are cutting all measurements in half because we can't afford to eat 2000 calories each day.
- Use canola oil for baking; olive oil for sautéing and broiling and coconut oil for frying.

Sodium – Scary in most prepared or processed foods. Mayoclinic.org reports:
- The benefits of sodium: maintains right balance of fluid in body; helps transmit nerve impulses and influences contraction and relaxation of muscles.
- Recommendation of 2,300 mg a day; but only 1500 mg a day if your age is 51 years or older, you are African-American or have high blood pressure, diabetes or chronic kidney disease.

It is my responsibility to recommend that you get your daily sodium requirements from your doctor and that you follow his/her instructions.

Making Eating Right Easy

Total Carbohydrates is the fiber and sugar in food.
Computing the amount of carbs in a serving is pretty simple.
- Your blood sugar goes up by 5 points times the sugar (carbs) count minus the fiber count. Example: Total carbs = 26. Subtract 5 fiber grams then multiply the remainder by 5. Math problem looks like this (26 – 5) x 5 = 105. That is a sure spike no matter how low your blood sugar is. If you eat right your blood sugar shouldn't drop below 80. If it does, you add 105 to the 80 blood sugar reading and you spike to 185! That is too great a rise. Your blood went from too thin to too thick. The train is chugging forward, perhaps pushing that car (clot) to your brain or heart!
- Sugar alcohol is present in most sugar-free or no sugar added products. Cut the total in half for a pretty accurate computation. Keep in mind a serving size on the label may not be a diabetic or hypertensive patient's serving size. Use your healthy plate chart.
- Fiber does not affect your blood sugar so it is not considered as something you need to be concerned about when it comes to controlling your blood sugar levels. However, fiber is extremely important. You want to eat 20 30 grams of fiber per day. Fiber cleanses your digestive track through the process of elimination (bowel movements).

Foods high in fiber include: whole wheat grains, whole wheat cereals, brown rice, vegetables and fruits, nuts, lentils. Serving sizes have to be adhered to so don't eat too much at one serving. The muffins in the recipe section of this guide are all high fiber foods.

Protein, vitamins and minerals are the last entries on the nutrition facts chart. Do read them.

Cynthia Bland

Essential Nutrients and the Foods That Provide Them

Vitamin A
- Aids vision (retina), skin and mucous membranes, teeth, soft and skeletal tissue and cell growth.

Foods that supply Vitamin A
- Cod Liver Oil (1 tbsp.) = Vitamin D and Omega 3 (fatty acids that lower triglycerides (a type of fat found in your blood) and blood pressure. Strengthens heart and possibly enhances mood. Get Vitamin A from your food. Supplements thin blood, so if you are taking blood thinners (anti-coagulants), it may cause bleeding. Ask your doctor about supplement use.
- Red pepper – fresh and dry (1 tbsp.)
- Oatmeal
- paprika (Vitamin C, potassium and calcium)
- Sweet peas
- Sweet potatoes 1 medium = 438% vitamin A daily requirement!)
- Kiwi
- ½ mustard and kale (Vitamin C, Vitamin E, Folate, Fiber, Protein and Calcium
- Carrots 1 medium = 200% of daily requirement (Vitamin C, K and B, magnesium, fiber)

Vitamin B group – Take B vitamin complex supplement and take once-a-day
- B12 - provides smooth functioning of body processes
- Converts carbohydrates into glucose which supplies ENERGY!

- ➢ Improves unhealthy cholesterol levels which protect against stroke and heart attacks
- ➢ Skin, hair and nail improvement
- ➢ Protects against breast, colon, lung and prostate cancers
- ➢ Regulates nervous system; reduces depression, stress and brain shrinkage

Foods that supply B vitamins
- ➢ Green peas, yams, broccoli, asparagus, turnip greens
- ➢ Peanuts, sunflower seeds, cashews, hazelnuts
- ➢ Whole wheat bread, cereals and bran
- ➢ Chickpeas, lentils, soybeans, kidney beans
- ➢ Fishes for vitamin B6: halibut, trout, snapper, salmon, tuna
- ➢ Milk, cheese, eggs, meat (turkey, chicken and pork loin (all white, low fat) and beef (good, low fat cuts)

Vitamin C
- ➢ Boosts HDL (good cholesterol that "drags" LDL (bad cholesterol) out of your blood) HDL is called lipoprotein that, perhaps, carries cholesterol away from your arteries and back to the liver where it passes from your body instead of sticking to the walls of your arteries causing a buildup of plaque prohibiting or stopping blood flow.
- ➢ Aids bone growth
- ➢ Aids growth and repair of tissue
- ➢ Collagen which supports tendons, ligaments and blood vessels

Foods that are rich in Vitamin C
- ➢ Kale
- ➢ Kiwi
- ➢ Red and green peppers

Cynthia Bland

- ➢ Broccoli
- ➢ Apricots
- ➢ Peaches

Vitamin D – The sunshine vitamin. 15 – 20 minutes 3x per week is sufficient.
- ➢ Vital to strong bones and teeth
- ➢ Vital to healthy immune system
- ➢ D3 – Great for the heart. I take 1000 International Units (IU) per day. My cardiologist approves!
- ➢ Found in beta cells that make insulin

Foods that supply Vitamin D
- ➢ Milk, vanilla yogurt
- ➢ Canned salmon, sardines and tuna, also catfish, and pork tenderloin
- ➢ Oatmeal, whole wheat and bran cereals, and grains
- ➢ Scallions
- ➢ 5 best cheeses in this order: Feta, Mozzarella, Parmesan, Swiss and Cottage. Avoid American cheese! It says processed right on label. Look at ingredients.

Iron
- ➢ Strength and energy
- ➢ Provides life-giving oxygen to organs through its role in red blood cell production
- ➢ Reduces cough and pre-dialysis anemia
- ➢ Regulates metabolism
- ➢ Vital source for healthy muscles

Foods that provide Iron

Making Eating Right Easy

- Blackstrap molasses which also provides B6, magnesium, calcium and antioxidants
- Spinach, green leafy vegetables, turnips, sprouts, broccoli, dry fruits
- Legumes (lentils, chickpeas, soybeans, beans and peanuts)
- Whole grains, cereals and bread

Good fats that enhance body's ability to absorb beneficial carotenoids which are: beta carotene, Vitamin A, Antioxidants, lutein and lycopene which strengthen bones, skin and immune function

- Almonds, walnuts, pistachios, peanut butter (limit to 2 tablespoons per day), seeds, nuts, grains, flax seed, dry roasted pecans (reduce triglycerides in blood)
- Coconut oil for cooking with high heat
- Fish oil is high in Omega 3 which reduces triglycerides in blood.
- Use olive oil for sautéing and salad dressings.
- Sardines, catfish
- Use Canola for baking

Fruit helps fight memory loss and improves cardiovascular health. While this is true, for diabetics and those attempting to lose weight (all diabetics and hypertensives with a waist line of over ½ the inches of your height) you must limit your intake. You can buy those wonderful parfaits that are packaged and sold in grocery stores and convenience store, but the ones you make yourself from scratch with fresh or frozen fruit and your homemade Granola (recipe included in this guide) are cheaper and safer to eat.

Fruit will satisfy your "sweet tooth" and supply fiber, vitamins and minerals that you need. You are to eat three meals a day and one snack between breakfast and lunch, and one snack between lunch and dinner. You can have ½ piece of fruit before bed along with a couple graham crackers with a smear of peanut butter on each to protect your blood sugar from dropping too low during the night.

- Papaya, kiwi, plantain (also vitamins and minerals)
- Guava, Asian pears and watermelon – high in lycopene, lowers risk of cancer and heart disease
- Star fruit – rich in Vitamin C
- Kumquats – essential oils (release oil by rolling fruit with fingers and then pop it, whole, into your mouth
- Cherries – contain a lot of sugar! Diabetics beware – limit serving.

- ✓ Anti-inflammatory – arthritic benefit and heart disease
- ✓ Anti-oxidant
- ✓ Provides melatonin – sleep aid
- ✓ High levels of potassium which aids in healthy blood pressure and quercetin which maintains vascular health

While meats, fish and poultry have nutritional benefits and just plain taste good, they contain cholesterol so you must limit your intake to 3 – 4 oz. servings. Meat can be eaten 2 days per week. Fish can be eaten 3 days per week. Because of the mercury in fish, pregnant women should limit themselves to 1 serving per week. Poultry (white meat) can be eaten 4 days per week. All of these foods should be broiled, baked or boiled. If you must fry, pan fry in coconut oil. Or use oven-fried method found in recipe section of this guide.

Making Eating Right Easy

Fat burners – slow digestion of carbohydrates burn slower throughout day. Helps curb appetite.
- Blueberries, avocado, broccoli, mushrooms and grapefruit. If you take blood pressure medication be sure to ask your doctor about grapefruit. Some counteract with your meds and can make you very ill. I don't eat grapefruit at all.
- Hot peppers, chili pepper flakes and ginger (fresh is best, if not use dry)
- Flax seed (1 tbsp. per day) use in yogurt, cereals, all baked foods, sauces, etc.
- Soybeans (edamame) – decreases appetite and builds muscles. Peanut butter, regular. Do not use low fat or other processes! Processed food is dangerous.
- Eggs – one for breakfast two times per week. They help lose significant baby fat.
- Green tea – burns belly fat. A couple tbsp. of Cider Vinegar in 8 oz. of water reduces inflammation and mucus.
- Olive oil – lowers bad cholesterol and improves cardiovascular health
- Walnuts and oatmeal keep blood sugar low
- Honey – encourages fat release from cells
- Water – 2 cups cold, boosts metabolic rate by 30%. 2 c. before breakfast, lunch and dinner = 17,900 calories per year (5 pounds lost).

Remedies for what ails you.
Joint Pain? Avoid fried foods, sugar, alcohol, carbonated beverages, grain-fed meat. Eat pineapple, kiwi, papaya, salmon, turmeric (a spice), walnuts and grass-fed meats.

Headaches? Eat flax seed – 1 tbsp. per day. Also spinach, mushrooms (which also raise metabolism) and asparagus.

Female concerns? Eat pineapple and almonds.

Heart concerns? Eat beans, nuts, take Vitamin. D3, Oatmeal, wild salmon (Omega 3), leafy greens, Swiss chard, kale, mustard greens.

Sleep concerns? Eat turkey, cheese (low-fat), raisins, 100% whole wheat bread (1 slice).

Offset sodium (blood pressure)? Sweet potatoes 3 x a week.

Liver ailments? Artichokes, commonly referred to as finger foods, contain potassium, Vitamin C, folic acid and have an abundance of antioxidants. The leaves of the artichoke contain cynarin and silymarin which boost liver function, boost regeneration of liver cells and decreases cholesterol levels which ward off arteriosclerosis (same as atherosclerosis, both vascular diseases). To make leaves palatable, put whole cooked leaf into your mouth then pull it out between your teeth to get the benefit of the nutrients inside the leaf.

Now we move to the scariest things in the world of health – the chemicals and additives that are put into our food. There have been many reports on the news broadcast channels that warn us of the addictive substances put in our food. These chemicals and additives are put in our food so that we will desire more and more of the food products in which they are contained. We wonder why a high percentage of this generation's children are

Making Eating Right Easy

overweight or obese. Well, wonder no more. It is a combination of the foods that they eat coupled with the ingredients in their food. Most fast food restaurants use the chemicals that addict our children.

The ingredients chart that follows includes many of the most commonly used dangerous chemicals and additives put in our food. It should scare you to death and make you commit to cooking from scratch. It should make fast food, eating out or commercially prepared pizza a once a month event.

Because I enjoy going to a restaurant, indulging in commercially prepared pizza and an occasional hot dog or sausage sandwich, I save my 5 to 6 teaspoons of recommended daily fat allowance for my "such a moment." But those moments occur less than once a month because I just don't want those poor blood test results. They do scare me! Literally scare me. Triglycerides, high LDL cholesterol – I don't ever want to "see" them swimming around in my blood again. And I won't because I choose to live an independent life right up to death's door. You can too.

My digestive disease physician's assistant, Ron Linquist gave me permission to use two quotes to get the point across: One is, "If the product you are contemplating buying is in the middle aisles of the store, don't buy it!" You will find some staples that you need in the middle aisles: grains, baking supplies, dried fruit, spices and herbs, kernel popcorn, pastas and a few others, but basically this is very sound advice. The other nugget he gave me is, "If it comes in a box or can, don't buy it." It is cheaper to eat right than to pay co-pays to be told to "eat right." What he is saying is what I have said, "Cooking from scratch is your best bet to insure that what you are putting in your system is going to benefit you."

Cynthia Bland

The other information mandated to be put on every food product is the ingredients that are put in edible products. This is another extremely important factor to consider if you really want to eat healthily. There are many dangerous chemicals that are put in edible products that do harm to your body organs.

One of the commercials that I really enjoy, because of how the point is driven home, is the Breyers ice cream commercial. Remember the young boy who couldn't pronounce the ingredients in other ice creams? Well, he could easily read the ingredients on Breyer's ice cream. Milk, sugar, cream, vanilla, etc. Pure products are what you want to purchase. My rule is if I can't read it, I don't eat it.

You don't have to memorize the following chemicals because this guide is published in pocket book size so that you can carry it everywhere you go.

Keep reading. You'll be amazed at the products that are chemically altered.

Making Eating Right Easy

Deadly Food Ingredients in the Food You Buy

The list of ingredients in a product is always in small print and there is no wonder why. I believe it is printed this way because the food producers don't want us, the consumer, to know all of their dirty little secrets about what they are serving us to put in our mouths.

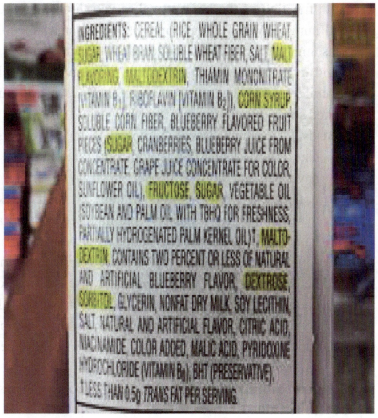

(gmofreegirl.com n.d.)

Cynthia Bland

The most dangerous chemicals put in your food are:

1. **Aspartame**: Nutrasweet and Equal – believed to be carcinogenic (cancer causing)
2. **High fructose corn syrup** – This is a manmade product. It packs on pounds, increases LDL (bad cholesterol), contributes to development of diabetes and tissue damage.
3. **Monosodium glutamate** – overexcites cells to point of damage or death, depression, disorientation, eye damage, fatigue, headaches and obesity. Because it affects the "I'M full" function of the brain it makes you think that you are still hungry. MSG is found in most chips, snacks, cookies, seasonings, soups, frozen dinners and lunch meats.
4. **Food dyes** – believed to contribute to behavioral problems in children and leads to reduction in IQ. Animal studies linked some dyes to cancer.

    Red dye #3, which has been banned in food products (to take effect when supplies run out), and Red dye #40 have been to thyroid cancer and may interfere with brain-nerve transmission. Found in fruit cocktail, maraschino cherries, cherry pie mix, ice cream, candy bakery products and many more foods.

    Blue dye #1 and #2 banned in Norway, France and Finland because they are believed to cause chromosomal damage. It is no wonder dyes have been banned. They contain titanium dioxide which is used in paint, sunscreen and food coloring! Found in candy, cereal, soft drinks, sports drinks and pet food.
5. **Sodium Sulfite** - causes breathing problems, rashes, headaches.
6. **Soduim nitrate/nitrite** – Turns old, dead meat bright red to give it the appearance of being fresh and vibrant. It is highly carcinogenic (cancer causing); wreaks havoc with

your pancreas and liver. Found in hot dogs, lunch meats, corned beef, smoked fish, bacon, ham and other processed meats.

7. **BHA and BHT** – preservative that keeps food from becoming rancid (Look at shelf life – noted on product "best used before ____"). Effects neurological system of brain, alters behavior and has the potential to cause cancer. Found in enriched rice, candy, jello, frozen sausage, potato chips and vegetable oil.
8. **Sulfur Dioxide** – Believed to cause bronchial problems, low blood pressure, destroys Vitamins B1 and E; avoid if you have emphysema, asthma or cardiovascular disease. Found in beer, soft drinks, dried fruit, juices, wine, some vinegars and prepared potato products.
9. **Potassium Bromate** – additive used to increase volume in some white flour, breads and rolls. Caused cancer in animals.
10. **Potassium sorbate**, calcium sorbate, sodium sorbate are all preservatives.
11. **Acrylamide** – Believed to be Carcinogenic. They are contained in the bag used for microwave popcorn.
12. **Acrylates – contained** in packaging of food products
13. **Titanium dioxide** – used as whitener in paint, food coloring, sunscreens, cosmetics, pigmentation for vitamins

Cynthia Bland

Substitutions for Deadly Food Products

Healthy foods that make high fat content, high sugar content a thing of the past.

For white wine:
- ➤ Chicken broth – Store-bought is expensive and high in salt and preservatives. Every time you boil chicken save the broth and use to cook veggies or for recipes that call for chicken broth.
- ➤ Water or white wine vinegar of red wine vinegar: dilute ¼ cup water per tbsp.
- ➤ Apple juice, white grape juice for sweet dishes. Dilute ¼ cup water per tbsp.

For sugar:
- ➤ ¼ cup honey for every cup of sugar. Reduce liquid by ¼ cup and increase baking soda by ¼ tsp. because honey produces excess liquid.
- ➤ Molasses – ¼ cup for every cup of sugar or your favorite sweetener. Be sure to use sparingly according to your taste. Cut liquid 1/3 cup and add 1 tsp. baking soda because molasses also produces excess liquid.

- ➤ Smart Balance seems to be the best spread to use instead of butter even though there is a great debate that suggests butter being better than any margarine or spread because butter will liquefy at room temperature and spreads, simply, don't. Coconut oil is also suggested for making grilled cheese sandwiches. I use pestos (recipes found in recipe section) as a spread instead of any of these, including mayo.

Making Eating Right Easy

- Sugar-free syrup for corn syrup (Never use high fructose corn syrup, it is man-made, therefore, a chemical) – There remains the question of sugar alcohol. The rule is: if the grams of sugar alcohol is less than the grams of sugar, go with the product with sugar alcohol. Count only ½ of the sugar alcohol calories/carbs as part of your daily intake.

- Fat free sour cream or fat free yogurt for toppings or recipes, yogurt instead of cream when baking dishes that call for milk.

- Fat free evaporated milk instead of half & half or heavy creams.

- Use fat free cream cheese.

- Use Red potatoes whenever possible. Red potatoes – New Potatoes have more Vitamin C, potassium, niacin and good carbohydrates and have less calories. You can bake or boil. Use your favorite spices and herbs to add excitement. White potatoes have a tad bit more thiamine, riboflavin, pantothenic acid, B6, iron and calcium than New Potatoes (red).

- Corn starch for thickening and binding ingredients instead of eggs or flour.

Chapter 2

Now Let's Shop

The Shopping Cart

I created a list for each of the recipes so that you can check to make sure you have all you need to prepare a good, healthy dish. Of course, you can always use your substitution list in this guide if you don't have exactly what the recipe calls for because a good cook always has the "perfect" ingredients to create a "perfect" dish.

I shop at Costco's or Sam's with two of my daughters for all items that I use frequently. Some of the fat-free products cannot be purchased at either of these food warehouses so I go to my favorite local grocery store to get them. By bulk shopping, you save loads of cash. Eating right is NOT more expensive than eating deadly dishes. We purchase paper toweling in large commercial packs and then divide them equally between the three of us (as we do the cost). We buy 10 gallon containers of dish detergent, laundry detergent and the 3-pack bleach and then fill up our individual dispensers. We spend on the average of $100.00 per person in each family per month and we eat and clean good!

The Pantry List

Herbs, Spices and Seasonings – I get the fresh bunches of most of my herbs, but keep the dried in case I run out. The herbs that are listed are the ones you will use frequently enough that you should buy the commercial sizes when available. What you can't get in commercial sizes you can find in the bins of grocery stores from $.88 to $1.00. I put an asterisk * next to each product that you will not find in food warehouses in bulk or commercial sizes.

1. Basil
2. Thyme
3. Parsley
4. Marjoram *
5. Turmeric*
6. Paprika
7. Ginger*
8. Garlic
9. Fennel which can be substituted with anise seeds *
10. Cinnamon
11. Nutmeg *
12. Ground cloves *
13. Bay leaves *
14. Sage
15. Organic salt-free seasoning
16. Italian Seasoning
17. Cayenne pepper
18. Ground and flaked red pepper *

Note: Black pepper is ground wood, so it is hard to digest. Cayenne heals the stomach as does red pepper, so they are preferred.

Sweeteners
- Honey
- Molasses – Blackstrap if possible *
- Home grown Stevia
- Splenda

Grains and Legumes
- Brown Rice, Couscous, or Quinoa *
- Oatmeal
- Cornmeal
- 100% whole wheat flour *
- Corn starch *
- Panko – Japanese bread crumbs – stay crispy longer than regular bread crumbs
- Ground flax seed – yellow or brown
- Pecans, walnuts and almonds
- Beans: kidney, pinto, white, Lentils *

Oils
- Olive oil
- Coconut oil
- Canola oil

Beverages
- Coffee
- Teas
- Water

Chapter 3

Now Let's Cook

I wrote the following recipes in a way that allows you to organize before you begin cooking. This way you can get all that you need, organize it so that you don't contaminate your refrigerator handles, cabinet knobs and other ingredients that you are not using for the recipe you are preparing. Salmonella can be deadly. You get and transfer it to others by allowing raw eggs, meat and fish to touch ingredients that are not going to be cooked to an internal temperature of 160 degrees or more. Wash your hands and all food preparation surfaces after touching raw eggs, fish or meat before preparing salads and fresh food side dishes.

Abbreviations used in this guide:
Ounce = oz.
Pound = lb. or #
Cup = c.
Teaspoon = tsp. or t.
Tablespoon = tbsp.
Quart = qt.
Gallon = gal.
Inch = "
Gm = gram
Mg = milligram

Cynthia Bland
Recipes

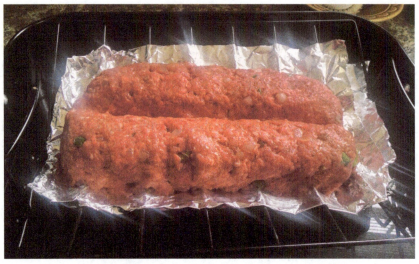

Veal Meat Loaf ready for the oven or grill

Recipe on page 69.

Making Eating Right Easy

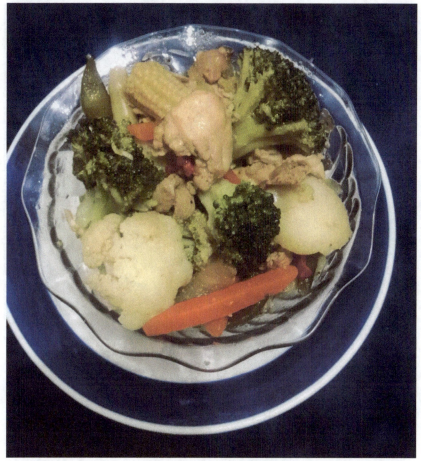

Stir fried chicken with Chinese vegetables and hoisin sauce

Recipe on page 58.

Hoisin sauce recipe on page 56.

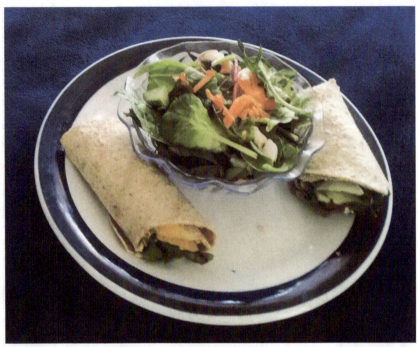

Chicken, Avocado, and Provolone Wrap with fresh greens and vegetable salad

Recipe on page 102.

Making Eating Right Easy

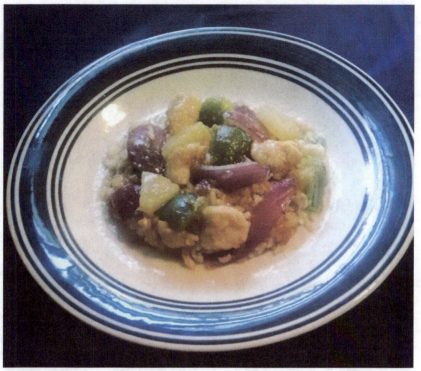

Sweet and sour pork tenderloin with purple onion, fresh mushrooms and green bell pepper

Recipe on page 59.

Cynthia Bland

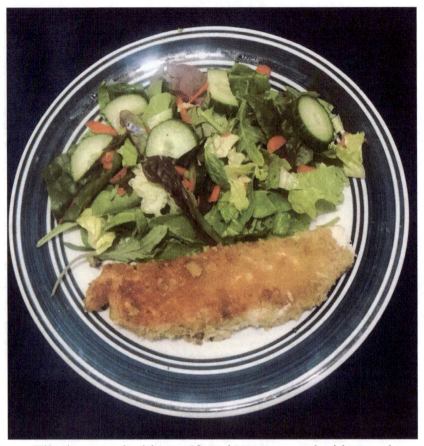

Tilapia crusted with your favorite nuts served with tossed vegetable salad

Recipe on page 50.

Making Eating Right Easy

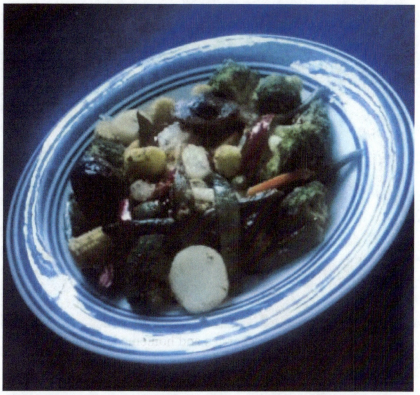

Roasted vegetables bathed in olive oil, spices and herbs, then oven roasted

Recipe on page 77.

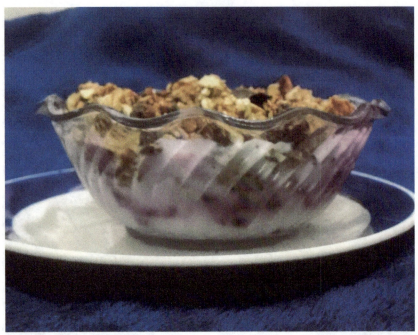

Plain Greek yogurt, blueberries and homemade granola parfait

Granola recipe on page 114.

Making Eating Right Easy

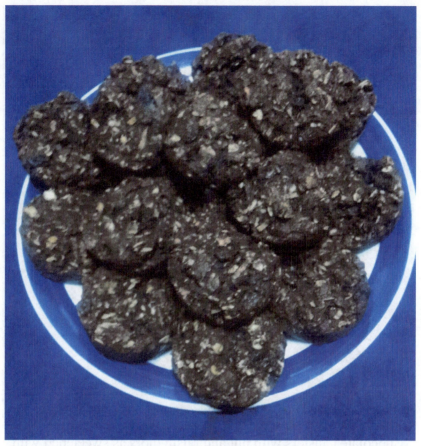

Use any muffin recipe and add ½ cup cocoa for these chocolate, oatmeal, nut and raisin muffins

Basic Muffin Recipe on page 115.

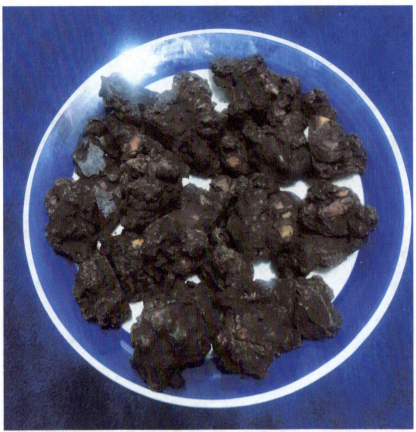

Chocolate Clusters with nut and raisin morsels sweetened with honey

Recipe on page 132.

Making Eating Right Easy

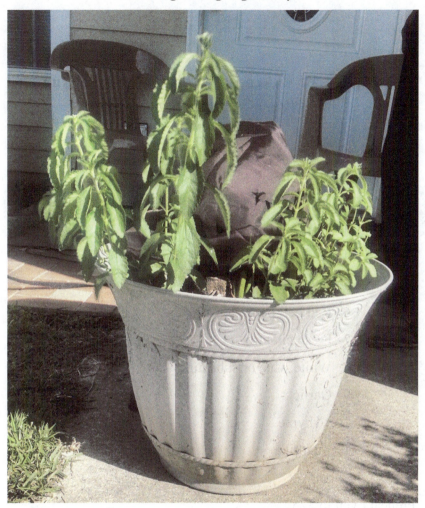

Grow your own sweetener – Stevia
Instructions for growing and harvesting on page 113.

Cynthia Bland

Healthy Entrees

Citrus Garlic Baked fish with Brown rice, quinoa (keen-uh-wah), or Couscous

Ingredients:
1. Four of your favorite fish filets
2. Rice, Quinoa or Couscous – enough to make 4 cups
3. Orange juice
4. Fresh lime or lemon
5. Red onion
6. Red bell pepper
7. Fresh cilantro
8. White wine or substitute
9. Garlic
10. Thyme
11. Paprika

Preheat oven to 325°
1. Cook rice, quinoa or couscous.
2. Place fish filets in baking dish, turning to coat with olive oil then arrange sliced red bell pepper and 1 cup fresh red onion slices over fish: sprinkle with 2 tbsp. coarsely chopped fresh cilantro.

Making Eating Right Easy

3. Combine ¼ c. white wine (or substitute), ¼ cup orange juice, 2 tbsp. fresh lime juice (I use lemon), 1 tbsp. minced or pressed garlic , 1 tsp. dried thyme (I use fresh.) and 1 tsp. paprika.
4. Pour mixture over fish. Bake uncovered 15-20 minutes or until 145° (flesh separates easily). Serve with grain of choice.

Serves 4. Calories 374; Total fat 3 gm (sat. fat 1 gm.); Cholesterol 99 mg; Sodium 136 mg; Potassium 1273 mg; Total carbs 31 gm. Fiber 5 gm; Sugar 6 gm; Protein 45 gm.

Pot Roast with Pinto Beans

Ingredients

1. Pot Roast
2. Diced fire-roasted tomatoes
3. Yellow onion
4. Garlic
5. Red, yellow and green pepper
6. Oregano
7. Chili powder
8. Cumin

9. Red pepper flakes
10. Pinto Beans, cooked

Preheat oven to 325°
1. Place meat in a baking pan.
2. Combine 14.5 oz. can undrained fire-roasted diced tomatoes, 1 small coarsely chopped yellow onion, 1 teaspoon pressed or finely chopped garlic, 8-oz. diced mixed red, yellow and green pepper (you can buy an 8 oz. bag in the frozen vegetables case), 1 tsp oregano, 1 tsp. chili powder, 1 tsp. ground cumin, ¼ red pepper flakes (hot! – be careful).
3. Pour mixture over meat. Cover with foil; bake 2-3 hours or until tender. When I got to this step the fat flag went up, so I cooked the roast until grease – not juice – drippings were in the bottom of the pan. I poured the fat off, took a few paper towels and removed all of the grease from the bottom and sides of the pan, then added mixture. Same result was achieved.
4. Add 1-15 oz. can fat-free pinto beans* (drained and rinsed) to roast.
5. Bake until beans are hot. Shred meat using two forks.

*I would plan my menu so that I would have leftover pinto beans cooked from scratch in my freezer – no preservatives or salt.

Making Eating Right Easy

Serves 4. Calories 306; Total fat 9 gm.; (sat. fat 3 gm) Cholesterol 60 gm; Sodium 1591 (if using canned beans and canned low salt broth. Prepare broth from scratch using no salt and this drops dramatically); Total Carbs 23 gm; Fiber 7 gm; Sugar 5 gm; Protein 25 gm.

Broccoli and Chicken Stir-Fry

Ingredients

1. 1 lb. boneless chicken breasts
2. Your favorite grain – 4 c. cooked
3. Garlic
4. Ginger
5. Red bell pepper
6. Low-sodium soy sauce
7. Orange juice
8. Chicken stock
9. 4 c. Broccoli florets
10. 1 medium-sized carrot
11. 1 medium-sized celery stalk
12. Canola oil
13. Olive oil

Cynthia Bland

1. Combine chicken (trimmed and cut into strips ¼" wide and 1" long), 1 tbsp. fresh ginger diced or pressed, 2 large cloves of garlic, peeled and minced, 1 ½ tsp. low-sodium soy sauce, ¼ cup orange juice and 2 tbsp. chicken stock. Set aside to marinate several hours ahead of cooking.
2. Steam 4 c. broccoli florets about 3 minutes (until bright green). Remove from heat.
3. In large pan, heat 1 tbsp. canola oil over medium-high heat. Add meat removed from marinade. Reserve marinade. Cook 1 minute.
4. In sauté pan, heat 1 tablespoon olive oil. When heated, add 1 red bell pepper cut into strips, 1 medium carrot and 1 stalk celery, both julienned. Cook 1 minute. Then add steamed broccoli florets and cook 1 minute more. If mixture gets dry add 1 tsp of oil. Cook another 30 seconds.
5. Add reserved marinade, along with ¼ c. stock and cooked chicken. Add more stock if more sauce is needed.
6. Stir and continue to cook another 1-2 minutes, until peppers, carrot, celery and broccoli are tender.
7. Serve with your favorite grain and enjoy.

Serves 4. Calories 235; Total fat 7 gm; (sat. fat 3 gm); Cholesterol 34 mg; Sodium 490 mg; Potassium 74 mg; Total Carbs 17 gm; Fiber 6 gm; Sugar 1 gm; Protein 25 gm.

Making Eating Right Easy

Roast Chicken with Green Beans and Artichokes

Ingredients
1. 1 3-4 lb. roasting chicken or 3-4 lb. skinned, defatted and boned chicken breast (much less fat)
2. 2 c. green beans
3. 2 fresh or frozen artichokes
4. 1 fresh lemon
5. Oregano
6. Onions
7. Garlic
8. Scallions
9. Parsley
10. Black and red pepper flakes
11. Olive oil
12. Chicken broth
13. White wine or substitute

Preheat oven to 400°.
1. Cut a 3 – 4 # chicken in half. Skin and de-fat. Lay the chicken, breast up, in baking dish. You can use skinned and defatted chicken breast, much less fat! It will cook faster saving you electric use. Yea! Adjust time if you choose to use breasts. Skin and defat your own poultry. It only takes a

few minutes and the little you throw away does not begin to add up to having the store do this at $7.00 per hour! Think smart and save money.

2. Arrange evenly on top of chicken: 1 tbsp. dried oregano, 1 tsp. black pepper, ½ tsp crushed red pepper flakes (Hot!), 4 coarsely chopped scallions, 8 cloves of garlic (crushed or pressed), 3 tbsp. olive oil.

3. When chicken starts to brown add ¾ cup white wine and ¾ cup chicken broth. (If canned, buy no fat, no salt).

4. Roast 10 minutes more then add 2 cups green beans, 1 cup fresh or frozen artichokes and 1 lemon sliced into ¼" rounds. Make sure the vegetables are submerged. Cook until tender about 10 minutes.

5. Garnish with ¼ cup chopped flat leaf parsley. Serve.

Serves 8. Calories 271; Total fat 7 gm (sat fat 1 gm); Cholesterol 82 mg; Sodium 149 mg; Potassium 222 mg; Total carbs 8 gm; Fiber 3 gm; sugar 2 gm; Protein 35 gm.

Pecan-Crusted Tilapia

Ingredients

    1. 5-6 pieces tilapia

    2. Buttermilk

Making Eating Right Easy

3. Whole wheat flour
4. Pecans
5. Grated parmesan
6. Garlic powder
7. Ground red pepper
8. Hot sauce
9. Canola or olive oil

In bowl #1 put: ½ c. Panko breadcrumbs, 2 tbsp. finely chopped pecans, 2 tbsp. grated parmesan, ¼ tsp, garlic powder and ¼ tsp. red pepper.

In Bowl #2 put: ½ cup buttermilk and 1 tsp. hot sauce.

In shallow dish put 3 tbsp. whole wheat flour.

1. Dredge each fillet in flour.
2. Dip in buttermilk mixture – shake off excess.
3. Dip in breadcrumb mixture – coat nicely.
4. In small frying pan put 1-½ tsp. oil (canola or olive oil).
5. Of the 6 – 8 fillets, fry only 2 pieces at a time on medium heat.
6. Fry 3 min. on each side or until fish easily flakes in middle when lifted by a fork.
7. Add 1- ½ tsp oil with each new 2 pieces.
8. Eat and enjoy this low fat wonderfully tasty dish.

Serves 6. Calories 122; Total fat 2 gm (sat fat 0gm; Cholesterol 57 mg; Sodium 58; Potassium 15 mg. Total carbs 4 gm; Fiber 0 gm; Sugar 0 gm; Protein 22 gm.

Spinach, Chicken and/or Shrimp, Mushroom Lasagna
(I prepared this with no meat or seafood – Delicious!)

Ingredients

1. Whole wheat lasagna noodles
2. Chicken breasts to equal 4 cups diced
3. 1 lb. shrimp
4. 1% milk or 2 cans fat-free evaporated milk
5. Parmesan cheese
6. 12 oz. bag spinach
7. 10 small mushrooms
8. Celery
9. Fresh garlic
10. Onion
11. Good olive oil "butter" spread

Preheat oven to 325°

1. Cook 12 whole wheat lasagna noodles.

Making Eating Right Easy

2. De-fat and skin enough chicken breasts to equal 4 cups diced (about two), then boil with 1 stalk celery, 2 cloves of fresh garlic, ½ small onion. (Remember to keep broth for future recipes).
3. Shell 1 # shrimp – do not cook!
4. Chop 3 cups fresh spinach and mushrooms.

White sauce: Alfredo

1. Melt 3 tbsp. good margarine.
2. Whisk in a bit at a time: 3 tbsp. whole wheat flour.
3. Add, stirring constantly – a bit at a time: 2 cups 1% milk.
4. Add 6 tbsp. of parmesan, 1 tsp. garlic powder (not garlic salt), a dash of red pepper flakes or ground red pepper.

Layer, in a pan that is the length of your cooked noodles. You will repeat this layering process 3 times.

1. Noodles.
2. Spinach and mushroom.
3. Chicken and/or shrimp.
4. Sauce - spoon on and spread.
5. Shredded parmesan cheese.
6. Cover with foil and bake at 350° for 1-1/2 hour.
7. Let set until firm.
8. Eat and enjoy this extremely healthy and tasty meal.

Cynthia Bland

Serves 12. Calories 231; Total fat 2 gm (sat fat 1 gm); Cholesterol 100 mg; Sodium 202 mg; potassium 418; Total carbs 27gm; Fiber 2 gm; Sugar 7 gm; Protein 24 gm

Alfredo sauce: Calories 127; Total fat 5 gm (sat fat 4 gm); *If you use shrimp, fat and sodium go up.

Risotto

Ingredients

1. 8 oz. shrimp
2. Arborio rice or brown rice
3. Mozzarella cheese
4. Chicken broth
5. White wine vinegar

Preheat oven to 325°

1. Sauté for about 3 minutes: 1 onion in 2 tbsp. olive oil and 1 pint of grape tomatoes (if too expensive, use diced plum tomatoes).
2. Add 1-1/2 Arborio rice (I use brown rice).
3. Stir in ½ c. white wine vinegar.
4. Cook until liquid has evaporated = 1 minute more.

Making Eating Right Easy

5. Stir in 4 c. chicken broth (frozen in your refrigerator) If you have to buy chicken broth buy low or fat-free, or use 2 cups chicken broth + 2 cups of water, or 4 cups of water.
6. Cover and bake 20 minutes to cook rice (brown rice takes a bit longer).
7. Stir in 8 oz. peeled and deveined shrimp and bake for 5 more minutes.
8. Remove, stir in 1 cup grated mozzarella cheese and 2 tbsp. healthy margarine.
9. Eat and enjoy.

For variety do same steps using 9 oz. crumbled Italian sausage, 1 sweet onion and 3 cups (5 oz.) baby spinach instead of tomatoes and shrimp. I cook my sausage and then use paper towels to press the grease – not juice – out of the meat. Paper towels are cheaper than the medical procedure or medication to remove the grease (cholesterol) out of your arteries and veins.

Serves 8. Calories 208; Total fat 10 gm (sat fat 4 gm); Cholesterol 61 mg; Sodium 498 mg; Potassium 112 mg; Total carbs 13 gm; Fiber 1 gm; Sugar 3 gm; Protein 15 gm.

Cynthia Bland

Pork and Mushroom Moo Shu

Ingredients
1. 1 lb. pork tenderloin
2. Shitake mushrooms
3. Chinese hot sauce or jalapeno
4. Low-fat soy sauce
5. Peanut butter
6. Molasses
7. White wine vinegar
8. Garlic powder
9. Sesame oil (or olive oil)
10. Black pepper or cayenne
11. Fresh ginger
12. Green onions
13. Broccoli slaw
14. Honey
15. Small corn or whole wheat tortillas

Because prepared foods are loaded with toxins (preservatives, salt, food colors), I cook everything from scratch ... hence

Hoisin Sauce: Mix until smooth: 4 tbsp. soy sauce (get low sodium), 2 tbsp. peanut butter, 1 tbsp. honey or molasses, 2 tsp white wine, 1/8 t. garlic powder, 2 t. sesame oil, 1/8 tsp. black

Making Eating Right Easy

pepper (I use cayenne) and 20 drops of Chinese hot sauce, or habanera, or jalapeno – not all three!

Preheat oven to 450°

1. Remove stems and slice 3.5 oz. shiitake mushrooms (or others).
2. Peel fresh ginger and grate/chop finely ½ tsp.
3. Chop coarsely ¼ cup green onions.
4. Cut 1 pork tenderloin (about 1 lb.) into four pieces – Wash hands!
5. Combine 3 tbsp. hoisin sauce, ginger and 1 tbsp. water.
6. Place pork in baking pan, pour ½ of hoisin mixture over pork and bake 8 – 10 minutes.
7. Whisk 3 tbsp. rice vinegar, 1 tbsp. agave nectar (or honey) and green onions until blended then stir in 12 oz. broccoli slaw. Let stand 8 – 10 minutes to marinate.
8. Add mushrooms to pork, bake 4 -5 minutes or until 160 ° in middle. Slice pork into thin strips then return to baking pan with mushrooms.
9. Stir in remaining hoisin mixture.
10. Microwave 8 small extra thin corn tortillas until thoroughly heated. If you don't have a microwave oven (good for you!) heat in oven until thoroughly heated or warm 1 at-a-time in a frying pan.

11. Top each tortilla with slaw and pork mixture. Serve and enjoy.

Serves 4. Calories 129; Total fat 4 gm; (sat. fat 1 gm); Cholesterol 27 mg; Sodium 139 mg; Potassium 230 mg; Total Carbs 13 gm; Fiber 2 gm; Sugars 3 gm; Protein 11 gm.

Hoisin sauce: Serves 4. Calories 23; Total fat 2 gm; Sat fat 0 gm; Sodium 53 mg; Potassium 1 mg.

Stir Fried Chicken with Chinese Vegetables

Ingredients
1. Chicken breasts
2. Olive Oil
3. Normandy Blend Vegetables – found in frozen food department
4. Cilantro
5. Oregano
6. Thyme
7. Tumeric
8. Red pepper flakes

1. Clean all fat and skin from 4 chicken breasts.
2. Dice chicken into 1" pieces.
3. Brown chicken in two tbsp. of Olive Oil.

Making Eating Right Easy

4. Remove chicken from pan and put in 4 cups of Normandy Blend vegetables.
5. Stir vegetables in chicken drippings until hot.
6. Sprinkle on top of vegetables: handful of chopped cilantro, teaspoon of oregano, thyme and ¼ teaspoon of turmeric. Add red pepper to your taste.
7. Add ¼ c. Hoisin Sauce.
8. Add diced chicken and stir until well-blended.
9. Eat and enjoy.

Serves 8. Calories 170; total fat 1 gm (Saturated fat 1 gm); trans fat 0; cholesterol 73 mg; sodium 65 gm. ; potassium 334 mg.; Total Carbs 4 gm; fiber 2 gm; sugars 2 gm; protein 24 gm.

Hoisin sauce recipe on page 56.

Sweet and Sour Pork Tenderloin with Purple Onion, Fresh Mushrooms and Green Bell Peppers

Ingredients

1. 1-1/4 lb. pork tenderloin
2. Brown Rice
3. Fresh Pineapple or large can pineapple chunks in its own natural juice

4. Pineapple juice from can of chunks
5. Sliced mushrooms
6. Fresh ginger
7. White vinegar
8. Low sodium Soy Sauce
9. Cornstarch
10. Catsup/Ketchup
11. Red Pepper flakes
12. Canola or Olive Oil

1. Cook rice – set aside.
2. In bowl, combine ½ c. Pineapple juice, 2 tbsp. white vinegar, 2 tbsp. low-sodium soy sauce, 2 tsp cornstarch, 1 tbsp. ketchup (negligible sugar source); and 2 tsp. finely grated fresh ginger or 1 tsp of powdered ginger.
3. In separate, bowl put fat-trimmed pork cut into 2" pieces. Sprinkle 2 tsp. cornstarch and ½ tsp. red pepper over it and then toss until pork is lightly coated.
4. Heat 1 tbsp. oil, add pork and cook until brown (about 5 minutes).
5. Take pork out of pan. In the drippings add: 1 green red pepper cut in 3" chunks, 8 oz. sliced mushrooms and 1 purple onion cut into 3" pieces – stir until crisp.
6. Stir into pan with green pepper and purple onion: pineapple chunks and pork.

Making Eating Right Easy

7. Whisk pineapple juice mixture then add to Pork mixture.
8. Cook on low heat until thickens. Serve and enjoy.

Servings 8. Calories 187; Total fat 7 gm (saturated fat 2 gm); cholesterol 47 mg; Sodium 164 gm; Potassium 436 mg. Total carbs 14 gm.; Fiber 1 gm; Sugars 10 gm; Protein 17 gm.

Add in from rice package the carbs in ½ cup. You don't have to eat this dish over rice.

Tomato-crusted Steaks over Vegetable Ragu

Ingredients

1. Tomato paste
2. Salt-free tomato basil seasoning
3. Balsamic vinegar
4. Zucchini
5. Onion
6. Tomato
7. Red bell pepper
8. 8 oz. portabella mushrooms
9. Paprika
10. Panko breadcrumbs

Preheat oven to 425°

Cynthia Bland

1. Whisk until smooth - 2 tbsp. tomato paste, 2 tbsp. water, 1 tsp. salt-free tomato basil seasoning and 1 tbsp. balsamic vinegar (Buy this vinegar. It is used a lot and has great nutritional value).
2. Toss with 1 medium zucchini, 1 small onion, 1 medium tomato and red bell pepper all cut into 1/2 inch pieces. Cut 8 oz. portabella (or others) in half.
3. Place vegetables on baking sheet in a single layer. Bake 15 – 20 minutes or until tender.
4. Combine 1 tsp. salt-free tomato basil seasoning, 2 tbsp. panko bread crumbs, 1 tbsp. grated parmesan cheese and ¼ tsp. ground paprika until blended.
5. Coat both sides of 1-1/2 pounds of grilling steak (filet, flat iron or top round) with bread crumb mixture (wash hands)
6. Place steaks on second baking sheet.
7. Bake 10 – 12 minutes or until 145° (for medium rare).
8. Serve and enjoy!

Serves 6. Calories 199; Total fat 7 gm; (sat fat 3 gm); Cholesterol 70 mg; Sodium 61 mg; Potassium 86 mg; Total carbs 4 gm; Fiber 1 gm; Sugar 1 gm; Protein 27 gm.

Making Eating Right Easy

Couscous-crusted Salmon

Ingredients
1. 4 Salmon steaks
2. Couscous or brown rice – 4 cups cooked
3. Lemon
4. Fresh parsley and basil
5. Raisins
6. Stuffed green olives
7. Pine nuts (I use walnuts – cheaper)
8. Canola oil

Preheat oven to 375° F
1. Grate 1 tsp. zest of lemon with NO white pulp – set aside.
2. Chop basil and fresh parsley coarsely to = ½ cup each. Place in medium bowl.
3. Stir into basil and parsley: 3 tbsp. raisins, 3 tbsp. sliced stuffed green olives, 2 tbsp. pine nuts (very expensive, substitute with finely chopped walnuts), lemon zest and ½ tsp. canola oil
4. Stir basil and parsley mixture into couscous.
5. Coat 9 x 13" baking dish with ½ tsp. oil. Add salmon, sprinkle with 1 tsp. salt-free tomato basil garlic seasoning.
6. Spoon couscous or brown rice evenly over fish and bottom of baking dish.

Cynthia Bland

7. Pour 2 cups water over couscous or brown rice.
8. Bake 20 = 30 minutes or until fish is 145° or until flesh separates easily. Squeeze lemon juice over fish.
9. Serve and enjoy.

Serves 4. Calories 378; Total fat 23 gm (sat fat 0 gm); Cholesterol 67 mg; Sodium 113 mg; Potassium 174 mg; Total carbs 37gm; Fiber 3 gm; Sugars 5 gm; Protein 28 gm.

Gumbo File

East Indians, French, Spanish and Africans tout this dish as a central part of their culture. West Africa's tout gumbo with okra as a cultural favorite.

You must follow these directions exactly as written. It is easy to burn the roux (rü or roo) which ruins the flavor of gumbo.

Roux – Use glass pot or wrought iron frying pan and wooden utensils. Roux will melt your plastic utensils.

Ingredients

      1. Your favorite sea foods: shrimp, whole crab claws, oysters, lobster

Making Eating Right Easy

2. 3 large chicken breasts
3. 1 lb. Kielbasa or other sausage (optional)
4. Canola oil
5. Flour
6. Bay leaves
7. Small onion
8. Fresh parsley
9. Pepper to taste
10. Olive oil
11. Green bell pepper
12. Red bell pepper
13. File (ground sassafras)

1. Put ¾ cup of oil in medium sized sauce pan, warm on medium heat then begin adding 2 tbsp. flour – a little at a time. GO SLOW! Do not scorch or burn – You'll have to start over. This is a 20 – 30 minute process of constant stirring. When it is a caramel colored brown, it is ready. Remove from heat.
2. Boil 3 quarts of water w/ 2 bay leaves, 1 small chopped onion, pepper to taste, 2 tsp. chopped parsley.
3. Add 1 lb unshelled shrimp, boil 2 minutes. Remove shrimp then devein and shell. Set aside. You have just made fish stock! Another stock that you can freeze for up to 6 – 10 months. No salt, preservatives, etc.

4. In clean skillet, sauté in 2 tbsp. olive oil: 1 small onion, chopped green and red bell pepper until soft.

5. Warm roux in large stock pot and strain shrimp stock into it. Slowly! Stirring gently.

6. Add sausage cut into 1" coins (I don't. Why add greasy meat to an otherwise healthy meal?)

7. Add sautéed and cubed chicken breast, 1 tbsp. thyme, parsley and pepper to taste.

8. Simmer 1 -2 hours.

9. Add shrimp, crab claws, oysters and/or lobster.

10. Cook slowly for a 3 – 4 minutes.

11. Add sassafras (1 – 2 tbsp. or to your taste).

12. Serve in soup bowl over rice. Really enjoy!

Serves 12. Calories 474; Total fat 10 gm (sat fat 2 gm); Cholesterol 254 mg; Sodium 949 mg; Potassium 598 mg; Total carbs 29 gm; Fiber 2 gm; Sugars 3 gm; Protein 65 gm.

Kale, White Bean, and Italian Turkey Sausage Soup

Ingredients

1. ½ lb. Italian turkey sausage
2. 1 qt. chicken stock
3. Olive oil

Making Eating Right Easy

4. Onion
5. Celery
6. Carrot
7. 8 c. kale
8. White beans
9. Bay leaf
10. Pepper
11. Parmesan cheese

1. Heat 1 tbsp. olive oil in large soup pot over medium-high heat. Add 2 sweet or spicy sausages cut into ½ "coins" and cook until browned. Remove sausage and set aside.
2. Add to the pot: 1 tablespoon olive oil. Lower heat to medium. Stir in c. diced onion, a large carrot, diced, and 1 large stalk of celery, diced. Cook until onion is translucent, about 8 minutes. Add 1 lb (about 8 cups) kale (ribs removed, leaves stacked and thinly sliced crosswise). Stir as they wilt and shrink down into the pot.
3. Add 2 cups pre-cooked white beans (If canned, rinse before adding to soup.), pepper to taste, 1 bay leaf, 1 quart of chicken stock and additional water, as needed, to cover.
4. Simmer soup for 15 minutes. Add sausage and simmer another minute.
5. Sprinkle grated Parmesan on top, if you desire.

Cynthia Bland

Serves 8. Calories 259; Total fat 9 gm (sat fat 8 gm); Cholesterol 39 mg; Sodium 1154 mg; Potassium 391 mg; Total carbs 27 gm; Fiber 9 gm; Sugar 3 gm; Protein 20 gm.

Sweet and Sour Chicken
(Pineapple is the only sugar source.)

Ingredients
1. 1-1/4 lb chicken
2. Rice
3. Fresh Pineapple or large can pineapple chunks
4. Pineapple juice
5. Fresh ginger
6. White vinegar
7. Soy sauce
8. Cornstarch
9. Catsup/Ketchup
10. Pepper
11. Canola or coconut oil

1. Cook rice – set aside.
2. In bowl combine ½ cup Pineapple juice (I get mine from the fresh pineapple.), 2 tbsp. white vinegar, 2 tbsp. low-

sodium soy sauce, 2 tsp. cornstarch, 1 tbsp. ketchup (sugar source), and 2 tsp. finely grated fresh ginger.

3. In bowl put 1-1/4 lb. skinned, boned and defatted chicken cut in 2" pieces w/ 2 tsp. cornstarch and ½ tsp. pepper.
4. Heat 1 tbsp. oil, add chicken and cook about 5 minutes (until brown).
5. Take chicken out and put on a plate. In the drippings add: 1 red bell pepper cut into 1" pieces – cook until crisp (about 2 minutes).
6. Stir into pan with red pepper: pineapple chunks and chicken.
7. Whisk pineapple mix #2 and chicken mix #3.
8. Cook until thickens. Serve and Enjoy!

Servings 8. Calories 187; Total fat 3 gm (sat fat 1 gm; Cholesterol 12 mg; Sodium 17 gm; Potassium 180 mg; Total carbs 33 gm; Fiber 3 gm; Sugars 6 gm; Protein 7 gm.

Veal Meat Loaf

Veal is not greasy, therefore a good choice of beef.

Ingredients
    1. 2 lbs. ground veal
    2. Breadcrumbs

3. Eggs
4. Carrot
5. Tomato sauce
6. Basil
7. Parsley
8. Thyme
9. Oregano
10. Chili powder
11. Milled flax seed – yellow or dark

Preheat oven to 375°

1. To 2 lbs. of ground veal add: 1 cup Italian bread crumbs (make my own by drying a couple slices of 100% whole wheat bread then crumbling it by hand or with a rolling pin.), 1 egg white – beaten, 1/3 cup shredded carrot (I tried with butternut squash – same result.), 1 c. tomato sauce with ½ tsp. of basil, ½ tsp. thyme or leaves of two stems of fresh thyme, ½ tsp. oregano, 1 tsp. fennel seeds or ½ tsp. ground fennel, ½ c. chopped onion, 1 tsp. dried parsley, ½ tsp. chili powder and ½ tsp. black pepper and ¼ cup milled flax seed.
2. Knead until thoroughly mixed then put in pan.
3. Bake covered for 45 minutes then uncovered for an additional 15 minutes.
4. Eat and enjoy!

Making Eating Right Easy

Serves 8. Calories 248; Total fat 10 gm (sat fat 3 gm); cholesterol 116 mg; Sodium 109 mg; Potassium 525 mg; Total carbs 13 gm; Fiber 2 gm; Sugar 2 gm; Protein 26 gm.

Chicken or Shrimp Alfredo

I used the lowest fat cheeses so my sauce was not velvety smooth. I didn't think to use my blender until after I'd put my shrimp in. You can try this method or just know that your Alfredo tastes great! Or you can use provolone instead of feta and mozzarella and put the parmesan on top of individual servings.

Ingredients

1. 12 oz. Fat-free evaporated milk
2. Corn starch
3. Mozzarella cheese
4. Feta cheese
5. Provolone cheese
6. Olive or coconut oil
7. Red pepper flakes
8. Ground red pepper
9. Parsley
10. Minced fresh garlic
11. Oregano

12. Thyme
13. 3 chicken breasts and/or 1 lb. shrimp
14. 1 Lb. fettucine
15. Parmesan

1. Pour 1- 12 ounce can of fat-free evaporated milk (12 oz.) + ½ can (6 oz.) into a sauce pot. Put on low heat.
2. Put 3 tbsp. corn starch in cold water and stir until dissolved.
3. Pour corn starch mixture into milk. Stir this mixture until it thickens (comes to slow boil).
4. Stir ¾ c. of shredded mozzarella cheese and ½ cup of crumbled Feta. Stir until melted. If you want to use your whole day's allotment of fat, use 1 cup of grated provolone. Remove from heat.
5. In medium sized frying pan, sauté in two tbsp. olive oil: ¼ tsp. red pepper flakes or a couple shakes of ground red pepper; 1 tsp. parsley.
6. 1 tsp. minced garlic or fresh pressed garlic; ½ tsp. oregano and ¼ tsp. thyme.
7. Add chicken to sautéed spices and stir until thoroughly cooked. If you are using shrimp, saute until pink.
8. Add sautéed mixture to sauce, stir until mixed.
9. Serve over linguine or fettucine cooked according to box directions.

Making Eating Right Easy

10. Sprinkle parmesan cheesed on top of each individual serving and enjoy.

Serves 8. Calories 289; Total fat 5 gm (Sat fat 1 gm); Cholesterol 26; Sodium 29 mg; Potassium 113 mg; Total carbs 42 gm; Fiber 2 gm; Sugar 2 gm; Protein 17 gm.

Alfredo Sauce. Calories 127; Total fat 5 gm (sat fat 4 gm) *If you use shrimp, fat and sodium go up.

Meatless Chili

Ingredients

1. Kidney or pinto beans
2. Large onion
3. Fresh garlic
4. Tomato sauce
5. Tomato paste
6. Chili powder
7. Cumin
8. Cilantro
9. Red pepper
10. Whole wheat spaghetti or macaroni (optional)

Cynthia Bland

1. Cook until soft: 1 lb. kidney or pinto beans (kidney beans are better for you) with 1 large diced onion, 3 pressed or diced cloves garlic.
2. While beans are cooking, pour 12 ounces tomato sauce and a small can of tomato paste into a small sauce pot.
3. Add to the tomato sauce mixture: ¼ c. chili powder; 2 tsp. cumin; handful of fresh cilantro or 3 tsp. of dried cilantro; crushed, flakes or powdered red pepper to taste. Let come to a boil, then stir and lower heat to low setting.
4. Let sauce reduce until beans are cooked.
5. When beans are very soft, stir tomato and chili spice mixture into beans and let simmer for ½ hour. Serve over whole wheat spaghetti or macaroni. If you must, sprinkle your favorite low-fat cheese on top.

Serves 12. Calories 167; Total fat 1 gm; Cholesterol 0 mg; Sodium 22 mg; Potassium 154 mg; Total carbs 34 gm; Fiber 6 gm; Sugar 4 gm; Protein 7 gm.

Making Eating Right Easy

Chicken Salad

Ingredients
1. Chicken breasts
2. Celery
3. Green pepper
4. Onion
5. Garlic
6. Pepper – black or white
7. Mayo made with olive oil

1. Skin and defat 2 large chicken breasts.
2. Put into enough water to cover chicken by at least 3".
3. Add to chicken: 2 stalks sliced celery, include leaves, 1 small diced onion, 3 cloves pressed or diced garlic.
4. Bring to boil, then put on low heat and let cook until cooked to the bone. No liquid at joint.
5. When thoroughly cooked, pour off water into a bowl or another pot. You are going to save this chicken stock for future use.
6. When chicken cools, pull chicken off bones. If you see any fat, cut it off and discard with bones.
7. Dice or shred chicken and put into medium bowl.

8. Stir into chicken: 2 stalks diced celery, ½ large diced green pepper, 1 tsp. parsley, red pepper flakes or ground red pepper to taste (optional), ½ tsp. marjoram, ¼ tsp. cinnamon and ½ tsp. oregano.
9. Add ½ c. reg mayo and ½ c. fat free mayo.
10. Clean sides of bowl with spatula, sprinkle paprika on top of salad – Enjoy!

Serves 12. Calories 108; Total fat 5 gm; (sat fat 0 gm); Cholesterol 0 mg; Sodium 136 mg; Potassium 58 mg; Total carbs 5 gm; Fiber 0 gm; Sugars 2 gm; Protein 11 gm.

Making Eating Right Easy

Healthy Vegetable and Grain Side Dishes

Roasted Vegetables

Ingredients

1. Normandy blend vegetables
2. Olive Oil
3. Powdered ginger
4. Oregano
5. Tumeric
6. Thyme
7. Garlic powder
8. Parsley – fresh or flaked
9. Paprika

Preheat oven to 400 degrees
1. Toss vegetables in 2 tbsp. Olive Oil.
2. Pour onto cookie sheet.
3. Sprinkle Oregano, turmeric, thyme, garlic powder, parsley and paprika over vegetables.
4. Place in oven. Let vegetable roast for 10 minutes then turn them over and roast another 10 minutes (until they are partially browned).

Cynthia Bland
Rotini Greek Salad

Ingredients
1. Whole wheat Rotini
2. Feta cheese
3. Walnuts
4. Red onion
5. Fresh spinach
6. Garlic
7. Dijon mustard
8. Pepper
9. White wine vinegar

1. Cook 8 oz. whole wheat Rotini – drain and chill.
2. Chop then toast ¾ c. walnut pieces over medium heat for 2 minutes. Stir as they toast.
3. In large bowl, toss chilled Rotini, walnuts, ¾ cup crumbled feta cheese, ¾ diced red onion and 2 c. chopped fresh spinach.
4. In small bowl, whisk 6 tbsp. walnut oil, 6 tbsp. red or white wine vinegar, 4 cloves garlic – pressed or minced, 1-1/2 tsp. Dijon mustard, pepper to taste.
5. Pour dressing over pasta, mix and toss.

Serves 4.   calories 364   Total fat 17 gm (sat fat 3 gm); Cholesterol 8 mg; Sodium 115 mg; Potassium 100mg; Total carbs 44 gm; Fiber 7 gm; Sugar 3 gm; Protein 12 gm.

Making Eating Right Easy

Stuffed Zucchini

Ingredients

1. Zucchini – 1 per 2 servings
2. Onion
3. Smart Balance margarine or
4. Turkey bacon
5. Fat-free sour cream
6. Roma tomatoes
7. Parmesan cheese
8. Curry powder
9. Thyme leaves
10. Pepper to taste

Preheat oven to 375°

1. Cut zucchini in half lengthwise, scoop out center.
2. Sauté 1 chopped large onion in 1 tbsp. "good margarine" until soft.
3. Fry 5-6 strips of turkey bacon until crisp. Chop into small pieces.
4. In separate bowl mix ½ tsp. curry powder, 2 tbsp. fat-free sour cream, 2 seeded and chopped Roma

tomatoes, 2 tsp. fresh thyme leaves, fresh grated ¼ c Parmesan cheese, pepper to taste.
5. Optional: chopped mushrooms and fresh garlic.
6. Mix all ingredients and stuff the zucchini shells.
7. Bake covered 30 minutes, then uncovered 10 minutes more.

Serves 4. Calories 131; Total fat 3 gm (sat fat 2 gm); Cholesterol 11 mg; Sodium 214 mg; Potassium 666 mg; Total Carbs 16 gm; Fiber 3 gm; Sugar 7 gm; Protein 7 gm.

Green Bean Casserole

Read whole recipe before preparing. You have to soak 3-1/2 oz. walnuts overnight.

Ingredients
1. Fresh green beans
2. Red onion
3. Mushrooms

Making Eating Right Easy

4. Quinoa
5. Flax seed
6. Flour
7. Sliced almonds
8. Walnuts
9. Skimmed milk
10. Reduced salt or salt free soy sauce
11. Tahini
12. Cayenne pepper
13. Canola and Olive Oil

Preheat oven to 350°

1. Top and tail 1 lb. of fresh green beans.
2. Steam for 3 minutes until bright green then **plunge into ice water,** drain and set aside.
3. Prepare topping: Separate sliced red onion into rings and toss in 1-1/2 cup quinoa flakes, 8 oz. sliced almonds and 1 tsp. marjoram.
4. Drain walnuts and blend with 1 tbsp. tahini, ½ c. skimmed milk, until smooth and creamy.
5. Heat tbsp. canola and 1 tbsp. Olive Oil over medium heat in heavy bottom sauce pan.
6. Add 2 minced cloves of garlic, cook 1 minute, then add ½ lb. sliced mushrooms, and ½ tsp. reduced or sodium free soy sauce, and ½ tsp. cayenne.

7. Toss continuously until mushrooms are soft and golden. Add1 tbsp. flour and 1/3 cup milled flaxseed and cook 1 more minute.
8. Add walnut mixture, ½ cup milk and 2 bay leaves – toss and stir gently.
9. When sauce is thick, add pepper and remove bay leaves.
10. Arrange beans in casserole dish, top with mushroom mix, then onion topping. Bake 20 minutes.

You can buy Tahini at an East Indian shop or make your own. Probably less expensive to buy ready-made if there are no dangerous chemicals added to the product. Read the ingredients label.

Preheat oven to 350°
1. Toast 5 cups sesame seeds for 5 – 10 minutes.
2. Toss frequently. Do not brown.
3. Put seeds into 1-1/2 c. olive oil and blend for 2 minutes.
Should be thick, yet pourable. It not, add a little oil.

Serves 8. Calories 330; Total Fat 14 glm (sat fat 1 gm).

Making Eating Right Easy

Sweet Potato Custard

Use in graham cracker crust for pie or just a wonderful side dish.

Ingredients
1. Sweet potatoes
2. Fat-free yogurt
3. Milled flax seed
4. Honey
5. Vanilla
6. Nutmeg, cinnamon
7. Pecans or walnuts

Preheat oven to 325°
1. Boil in just enough water to cover - 4 large sweet potatoes cut into 4ths (saves electric or gas).
2. When very soft, drain, peel and put in large bowl.
3. Mash until smooth, then whisk until smooth (blend if you have a blender).
4. Add ¼ cup milled flax seed, 2 cups fat free yogurt, 1/2 c honey, 2 tsp. vanilla, nutmeg, cinnamon and 1 cup finely chopped pecans.
5. Bake until as firm as you like.

Serves 8. Calories 213; Total fat 6 gm (sat fat 1 gm); Cholesterol 14 mg; Sodium 111 mg; Potassium 365 mg; Total Carbs 39gm; Fiber 3 gm; Sugar 23 gm; Protein 6 gm.

Cynthia Bland

Pan-Fried Quinoa Cakes

Quinoa (pronounced keen-wah) is a grain that you find at your local grocery in the aisle that has special/unique grains. It comes flaked and granulated. It is a great substitute for white rice as is couscous, barley and brown rice. Quinoa lowers cholesterol, has 15% fewer carbs, 60% more protein than brown rice, 25% more fiber than other grains and it lowers cholesterol.

I had a hard time getting this mixture to bind, so I formed the patties with a ¼ c. measuring cup, placed them on a cookie sheet and froze them before frying. Worked like a charm.

Ingredients

1. Quinoa
2. Kale
3. Sweet potatoes
4. Eggs
5. Milled flax seed
6. Yellow onion
7. Parmesan cheese
8. Fresh dill

Making Eating Right Easy

9. Cayenne
10. Olive oil

1. In a large pot, bring 4 c. water to boil, add ½ pound of kale (stems removed and chopped. Cook 1 minute then scoop out into a large bowl, reserving cooking water.
2. When kale is cool, squeeze out excess water; set aside.
3. Bring reserved water back to a boil and add ¾ cup peeled and diced sweet potatoes. Simmer until crisp-tender about 3 minutes. Scoop potatoes into a bowl, set aside, reserving cooking water.
4. Measure out 3 cups of cooking water, discard the rest, then pour the 3 cups back into the pot. Bring water to a boil, add 2 cups rinsed and well-drained quinoa and stir. Reduce heat to medium-low, cover pot and simmer until water is absorbed, about 12 minutes. Stir in ¼ cup of milled flax seed. Remove from heat and set aside, covered for ten minutes.
5. Add quinoa to bowl of kale and toss to combine. Gently mix in sweet potatoes, 1 small diced finely yellow onion, ½ cup finely grated Parmesan cheese, 2 tbsp. minced fresh dill, ¼ tsp. cayenne. Set aside to cool 10 minutes. Add 4 large eggs (2 whites + 2 whole) or (4 whites), mix to combine.

6. Using a ½ cup measure, scoop quinoa mixture, press firmly to level the tom, turn cup over on baking sheet. Make 14 patties.
7. In large skillet, heat 2 tbsp. Olive oil over med head. Cook 4 – 6 patties at a time. Carefully flip the cakes after golden brown, and brown the other side. About 4 minutes longer. Add more oil, as needed, to cook additional batches.
8. Serve with creamy yogurt and dill sauce.

Serves 16   Calories 180; Total Fat 10 gm (sat fat 2 gm); Cholesterol 3 mg; Sodium 78 mg; Potassium 295 gm; Total carbs 19 gm; Fiber 2 gm; Sugar 1 gm; Protein 6 gm

The next few recipes are oven fried delights. If you love crispy foods, these will satisfy you. Much lower in calories and fat, yet crispy finger foods.

Chipotle Cornmeal Green Bean Fries

Ingredients
1. Fresh green beans
2. Buttermilk
3. Cornmeal

Making Eating Right Easy

    4. Chipotle chili pepper

    5. Honey

Preheat oven to 475°

1. Bring a pot of water to a boil. Have a bowl of ice water ready.
2. Add green beans to pot and cook 2 minutes; transfer to ice water 2 minutes then put on kitchen towel and blot dry.
3. Place a rack in the lower third of the oven and a second one in the center.
4. In a large bowl, mix together 1 c. buttermilk, 1 tsp. ground chipotle chili pepper, 1/4 c. honey, and ½ cup cornmeal. Set aside 10 minutes.
5. Toss beans in buttermilk mixture to coat.
6. Arrange, without crowding, in a single layer on baking sheets or wire racks.
7. Bake until coating is golden and crisp – 8 – 10 minutes.

Serves 4. Calories 161; Total fat 1 gm (sat fat 0 gm); Cholesterol 2 mg; Sodium 74 mg; Potassium 262 mg; Total carbs 36 gm; Fiber 3 gm.

Cynthia Bland

Carrots Garam Masala

Garam Masala is an Indian spice blend of: cinnamon, red pepper, cumin and ground cloves. Because I enjoy this spice blend, I make a large amount and store in used shaker bottles. 6 tbsp. cinnamon, 1 tsp. red pepper, 2 tsp. cumin and 1 tsp ground cloves. Make your own for less money.

Ingredients

1. For Garam Masala: cinnamon, cloves, red pepper, cumin
2. Carrots
3. Rice flour (or wheat)
4. Canola oil

Preheat oven to 450°

1. Arrange rack as you did for the Green Bean Fries.
2. Line rimmed baking sheets with parchment paper – I will oil mine.
3. Cut 2 lbs. large carrots into French fry size sticks = 3" long.
4. In a large bowl, toss carrots with rice flour to coat.
5. Shake off excess flour and spread carrots without crowding in a single layer on baking sheets. Bake 7 minutes.
6. Combine 6 tbsp. canola oil and garam masala. Gently toss carrots.

7. Return carrots to pan and bake until crisp tender and lightly browned along edges. 10 – 15 minutes.

Serves 4. Calories 353; Total Fat 22 gm (sat fat 2 gm); Cholesterol 0 mg; Sodium 48 mg; Potassium 254 mg; Total carbs 38 gm; Fiber 3 gm; sugar 3 gm; Protein 3 gm.

Spiced Sweet Potato Fries

Ingredients

1. Sweet potatoes
2. Canola oil
3. Cajun/Creole seasoning (see: Cajun/Creole Mayo recipe)
4. Splenda, if necessary for sweeter dish

Preheat oven to 450°

1. Arrange racks, baking sheets and cut potatoes as you did carrot masala.
2. In a large bowl, mix ¼ c. canola oil, 1-1/4 tsp. Cajun/Creole seasoning.
3. In a large bowl, mix ¼ c. canola oil, 1-1/4 tsp. Cajun/Creole seasoning and 1/2 tsp. Splenda. Only use Splenda if potatoes are not sweet enough for you.

4. Toss potatoes to coat.

5. Place in single layer on prepared sheets. Bake 15 minutes, flip over and continue to bake until crisp-tender and nicely browned at the edges. About 10 -15 minutes longer.

Serves 4.   Calories 204; Total Fat 14 gm (sat fat 1 gm); Cholesterol 0 mg; Sodium 54 mg; Potassium 329 mg; Total carbs 20 gm; Fiber 3 gm; Sugar 4 gm; Protein 2 gm.

Oven-baked Steak Fries

Ingredients
1. Red or white potatoes
2. Canola oil
3. Pepper

Preheat oven to 475°

1. Follow steps for garam masala carrots, except cut potatoes in half lengthwise and then cut each half into 6 long wedges.
2. Submerge potatoes in large bowl filled with hot water and soak for 10 minutes.
3. Drain, rinse, and pat dry with paper towels.
4. Toss potatoes with ¼ c. canola oil and 1 tsp. pepper.

Making Eating Right Easy

5. Arrange in single layer. Cover each pan tightly with aluminum foil; bake 5 minutes; remove foil; bake 15 minutes more.

6. Flip potatoes and rotate pans, then bake until browned and crisp at the edges, about 10 – 15 minutes more.

Serves 4. Calories 404; Total fat 14 gm (sat fat 1 gm); Cholesterol 0 mg; Sodium 22 mg; Potassium 1553 mg; Total Carbs 64 gm; Fiber 8 gm; Sugar 3 gm; Protein 7 gm.

Parmesan Zucchini Fries

Ingredients

1. Fresh zucchini
2. Flour
3. Parmesan cheese
4. Dill (optional)
5. Panko or regular breadcrumbs
6. Egg whites

Preheat oven to 425°

1. Follow steps as in Garam Masala carrots, except cut 1-1/2 pounds zucchini as you did the potatoes but only 3" long.

2. Arrange 3 shallow pans in a row. In first bowl, stir together ½ c. flour, ½ tsp. ground black pepper. In the second bowl, whisk together 3 egg whites and ½ tsp. ground black pepper. In the third bowl combine 1-1/2 panko crumbs (or your own), ½ cup Parmesan cheese and 1 tbsp. dill (optional).
3. Working in batches, first dip zucchini in flour, shaking off excess. Transfer to egg mixture and toss until coated. Let excess egg run off, then coat zucchini in panko or breadcrumb mixture.
4. Arrange zucchini in a single layer, bake 15 minutes and then rotate the pans. Continue to bake until panko coating is golden and crisp about 7 – 12 minutes longer.

Serves 4. Calories 305; Total fat 6 gm (sat fat 2).

Pepper Slaw

Ingredients
1. Green cabbage
2. Red cabbage
3. Carrots
4. Scallions (green onions) (optional)
5. Rice vinegar

Making Eating Right Easy

6. Hot pepper vinegar
7. Molasses
8. Sesame oil (Olive oil is better)
9. Sesame seeds or your favorite nuts chopped very fine – I use walnuts because they are an integral part of my healthy diet.

1. Discard the outer leaves of the medium head of green cabbage and the small red cabbage.
2. Peel and grate into thin shreds, 3 large carrots.
3. Drain off any liquid produced by the cabbage.
4. Add carrots to cabbage and mix well.

Dressing: Whisk 1/3 c. rice vinegar, 1/3 cup hot pepper vinegar, ¼ cup light brown sugar (molasses would be healthier choice, but just a tablespoon. and 1-1/2 tbsp. dark-roasted sesame oil.

1. Pour dressing over cabbage mixture and mix well.
2. Garnish with ¼ c. minced scallions and 1 tbsp. toasted sesame seeds before serving.

Serves 8. Calories 54; Total fat 0; Cholesterol 0 mg; Sodium 51 mg; Potassium 526 mg; Total carbs 13 gm; Fiber 5 gm; Sugar 8 gm; Protein 3 gm.

Cabbage dressing: Calories 43; Total fat 3 gm (sat fat 0 gm); Cholesterol 0 mg; Sodium 282 mg; Total barbs 4 gm; Fiber 1 gm; Sugar 2 gm   *Remember to add the values for total nutrition facts.

Chicken Vegetable Soup

Ingredients
1. Three Chicken breasts
2. Olive oil
3. Celery
4. Carrots
5. Green beans
6. Tomatoes
7. Cilantro
8. Parsley
9. Oregano
10. Marjoram
11. Turmeric
12. Brown rice, quinoa, couscous or whole wheat pasta (These are all optional. Because we must do low carbs, I serve my soup with salt-free whole wheat crackers)

The nutrients chart that follows the recipe does NOT include a calculation of any grains. If you add a grain, go to google and

Making Eating Right Easy

type in carbohydrates in ½ cup of grain choice to get an accurate carb count.

1. Put 2 lbs. skinned and defatted chicken breasts in cold water that is 3" above meat
2. Bring to a boil, then reduce to medium heat and cook until done (There is no blood on or near bone)
3. Remove chicken from water and place on plate to cool
4. Dice 4 stalks of celery, 8 carrots, 2 large tomatoes, 4 cups string beans, tips cut off and cut into bite sized pieces
5. Sauté in 1 tbsp. of olive oil for 5 minutes: vegetables, 5 sprigs of chopped cilantro and 4 sprigs of chopped parsley, 1 teaspoon of each: oregano, marjoram and turmeric.
6. De-bone and dice chicken breast
7. Skim water with spoon and paper toweling to remove any excess fat
8. Put all vegetables, spices, herbs and chicken back in water. Bring to a boil, then reduce heat to simmer.
9. Simmer soup until the liquid is reduced to your taste.

Serving size 1 cup; Calories 167; Total fat 3gm (sat fat 1gm); Cholesterol 65 mg; Sodium 248mg; Potassium 230 mg; Total Carbohydrate 10gm; Fiber 3gm; sugars 4gm.

Cynthia Bland

Lentil Soup

I love chicken soup, but I love lentil soup more! It has great nutritional benefits and taste really great. The lentils do not require soaking, so this is listed as a quick fix. Put them on at 5:00 pm; they are ready in about 45 minutes.

Ingredients

1. 1 bag lentils
2. 1 lb. Chicken or turkey sausage if you must have meat or fresh Italian sausage
3. Fresh carrots
4. 1 medium onion
5. Fresh celery
6. Pepper to taste
7. Basil
8. Oregano
9. Thyme

When I prepare lentils, I do not add meat, especially prepared or preserved. I would add 1 diced chicken breast or cooked, defatted fresh Italian sausage to satisfy those who cannot forego meat. It is a fact that the meat taste like the lentils. You couldn't tell whether there is meat in the soup if you were blindfolded.

Making Eating Right Easy

1. Rinse 1 lb. of lentils in pot of cold water. Pour off water, add fresh water to 2" over lentils. (You may have to add a little water if the soup cooks down and becomes thick).
2. Brown meat and absorb fat with many paper towels. Press and squeeze meat until the paper towel is free of fat.
3. Put 3 diced carrots, diced onion, and diced celery into pot along with spices.
4. Bring to boil over high heat. Reduce heat to low and cook for 35 minutes.
5. Add cooked meat.
6. Reduce heat to low and let simmer until ready to eat. About 15 minutes.

Serves 8. Calories 242 Total Fat 1 gm (sat fat 0 gm) Cholesterol 0 mg; Sodium 15 mg; Potassium 801 mg; Total Carbs 43 gm; Sugars 5 gm; Protein 18 gm.

Basic Tossed Salad

I eat a large salad almost every day even when I have vegetables planned on my daily menu. Sometimes I just eat a large salad topped with my favorite things. It is truly a good, healthy meal and filling. You do have to consider all of your toppings.

Remember, some have carbohydrates. Some have fat (avocado is one – but it is a healthy fat).

1. Shred 1 cup of any leaf lettuce (red leaf, green leaf or iceberg lettuce), 1 cup of fresh kale, 1 cup Swiss Chard, ½ cup arugula. Mix the greens by hand or toss with large fork.
2. Dice ¼ of each: red bell pepper, yellow bell pepper, orange bell pepper. Sprinkle the peppers on top of salad. Really pretty! Chop scallions, to taste, and sprinkle on top.
3. Choose toppings: 1 chopped boiled egg, ¼ cup raisins, 2 tbsp. of crumbled feta cheese, chopped black or green olives, sliced mushrooms. There are other toppings that you might enjoy. Leave some out or add others. Just make sure you don't overdo the cholesterol (egg and cheese) or fat (avocado and cheese) or carbs (carrots).
4. Serve with olive oil and vinegar or a store bought vinaigrette made with olive oil. I also enjoy the raspberry dressings. Count the sugar and fat if you use store bought dressings.
5. I sometimes enjoy no-salt top crackers with my salad or a slice of toasted whole wheat bread.

Making Eating Right Easy

Sandwiches and Quick Fixes
Pan-Fried Pizza

This pizza is healthier than any you can buy because you control the preparation of the toppings that you choose. Have plenty of paper towels to drain and squeeze out grease – NOT juice! - of any meat and to absorb oil off the cheese when it comes out of the pan. You will see oil sitting on top! Don't get confused, you are not getting rid of flavor, just grease! Loss of flavor – what an excuse to pack those arteries and veins hm-m-m! And don't forget about your poor liver. Don't work it so hard!

Ingredients
1. Pizza dough
2. Tomato sauce
3. Mozzarella
4. Fennel seeds
5. Oregano
6. Basil
7. Your favorite pizza toppings

Preheat broiler
1. Divide store-bought pizza dough in half. Working with one piece at a time, roll or stretch out each piece into 10" – 12" rounds. As big as your largest ovenproof skillet.

2. Pour enough olive oil into the large skillet to thickly coat bottom of pan, about 1/8" thick. (Olive oil is good fat).
3. Heat pan on medium high until oil starts to shimmer.
4. Place 1 round of dough in pan and cook until bottom is crisp and browned, being careful not to let it burn, about 3 minutes.
5. Flip over dough and top browned side with ¼ cup of tomato sauce, 4 – 6 oz. mozzarella, 1 tbsp. fennel seeds, 2 tsp. oregano leaves or powder and 8 – 12 basil leaves. Here is where you can add sliced tomatoes, zucchini, onion, green pepper, olives, etc. You can even add meat – Just make sure you absorb all of the grease that is possible.
6. When bottom is browned, transfer pan to oven until cheese begins to melt, 2 minutes. Remove from oven and make second pizza.

Serves 4. Calories 345; Total fat 5 gm (sat fat 3 gm); Cholesterol 18 mg; Sodium 425 mg; Potassium 1053 mg; Total Carbs 53 gm; Fiber 8 gm; Sugar 12 gm; Protein 17 gm.

Making Eating Right Easy

Avocado Sandwich
My favorite sandwich

Ingredients
1. Avocados
2. Red onion
3. Mayo
4. Bell pepper

1. Lay two slices of whole wheat bread side-by-side on your plate.
2. On one slice of bread spread ½ fresh ripe avocado.
3. On the slice piece spread Smart Balance Mayo and relish or pickle of your choice.
4. On top of the avocado, place a couple rings of red onion, then top that with thin strips of red, green, yellow or orange bell pepper.
5. Close the sandwich and eat to your heart's delight!

Serves 1. Calories 353; Total fat 14 gm (sat fat 1 gm)

Cynthia Bland

Chicken, Avocado and Provolone Wraps

Ingredients
1. Chicken breast
2. Avocodos
3. Sliced provolone*
4. Your favorite lettuce
5. Tomatoes
6. Cilantro
7. Hot pepper sauce
8. 10" tortillas

*I used Swiss cheese because it has more calcium than Provolone.

1. Combine in a bowl: 2 cups shredded or chopped cooked chicken (Remember to save broth!), ½ cup chopped tomato, ¼ cup chopped cilantro, ½ tsp. hot pepper sauce, and toss well.
2. Add 1 diced avocado; toss again.
3. Arrange 4 slices provolone cheese over tortillas; top with red leaf lettuce or Boston lettuce leaves.
4. Roll up; cut each roll diagonally.

Serves 12. Calories 270; Total fat 12 gm; (Sat. fat 4 gm); Cholesterol 40 mg; Total Carbs 28 gm; Fiber 5 gm.

Making Eating Right Easy

Turkey Burger

Ingredients
1. Ground turkey
2. Paprika
3. Cumin
4. Pepper
5. Milled flax seed

1. Mix and form 4 – 4" patties with: 1 lb. ground turkey, 1 garlic clove pressed/minced, ½ tsp. paprika, ½ tsp. ground cumin, ¼ tsp. pepper and ¼ c. milled flax seed.
2. Grill until thoroughly cooked – 7 minutes on each side.

Serves 4. Calories 223; Total fat 13 gm (sat fat 3 gm); Cholesterol 84 mg; Sodium 88 mg Potassium 221 mg; Total carbs 2 gm; Fiber 2 gm; Sugar 0 gm; Protein 24 gm.

Toppings to make turkey burgers utterly delicious:
1. Spicy Blue burger: 3 oz. bleu cheese, sliced and 2 tsp. ketchup mixed with hot sauce to taste.
2. California: 1 avocado sliced, ¼ c. tomatillo salsa.
3. BBQ: 4 slices sweet onion, ¼ c. BBQ sauce.

Cynthia Bland

Salmon Burgers

Ingredients
1. Fresh salmon
2. Panko or regular breadcrumbs
3. Flax seed
4. Pepper
5. Egg white

1. Pulse or chop finely – remove all bones 1 lb. skinless salmon.
2. Add ½ cup panko breadcrumbs and ¼ cup milled flax seed, ½ tsp. pepper and 1 large egg white and chop until fine.
3. Form 4 – 4" patties.
4. Grill 5 – 7 minutes each side.

Serves 4. Calories 198 Total fat 7 gm (sat fat 1 gm); Cholesterol 91 mg; Sodium 295 mg; Potassium 18 mg; Total Carbs 12 gm; Fiber 2 gm; Sugars 1 gm; Protein 24 gm.

Bun Choices:
1) Toasted Ciabatta (BBQ)
2) Toasted brioche (California)
3) Toasted sesame seed (BBQ)

Making Eating Right Easy

Healthy Dips, Dressings and Sauces

Ranch: 4 slices tomato, grilled. ¼ c. ranch dressing non-fat! Serve on toasted Brioche bun.

Asian: 3 tbsp. fat-free mayo + 1 tsp. low sodium soy sauce, ¼ cup scallions. Serve on toasted sesame seed buns.

Greek: ½ cucumber slices, ¼ cup crumbled feta. Serve on toasted ciabatta rolls.

Dips
Lemony Yogurt Dip with Dill:
Whisk: 1 c fat free yogurt, 2 finely minced garlic cloves, 2 tbsp. finely minced dill, 3 tbsp. lemon juice, 1 tsp. lemon zest, and ¼ tsp. black pepper.

Quick, creamy sauce: Mix Greek-style yogurt with chopped dill, lemon juice and salt to taste.

Cynthia Bland

These dips can be enjoyed for taste, nutritional value and healthy fat and sugar levels; they are low to no fat and low to no sugar! Make from scratch! Healthier, no added salt, preservatives, etc. What you pay $4 - $5 for prepared product; you get for pennies per serving.

You can use these pestos in pasta and shrimp salads; pasta and chicken salads or on sandwiches instead of mayo. They are extremely healthy and other than the natural fat, salt, and fructose or sucrose in the plants, we added NONE!

Basil Pesto

Puree or pulse 1 c. fresh basil, ½ c. parmesan cheese, ½ c. olive oil and 1 -2 cloves of garlic. That's it!

Double the recipe and freeze ½ cup servings in small sandwich bags then put in 1 large gallon storage bag. Freeze for up to 6 months.

Spinach Pesto

Pulse or puree 4 c. fresh torn spinach, 3 cloves garlic, 3 tbsp. pine nuts (expensive! I use walnuts), ½ tsp. dried basil, ¼ cup olive oil or walnut oil and 1/3 c. parmesan cheese. That's it!

Making Eating Right Easy

Put 1 cup servings in sandwich bags, then put all of the bags in a gallon storage bag and freeze for up to 6 months.

Serves 8. Calories 173; Total fat 10 gm (sat fat 1 gm); Cholesterol 2 mg; Sodium 112 mg; Potassium 1082 mg; Total carbs 21 gm; Fiber 7 gm.

Cheese Pepperoncini

(substitute w/ banana pepper; Hot or Mild)

1. Blend ¼ c. fat-free sour cream and 2 tbsp. fat-free cream cheese until smooth.
2. Add 1 c. fat-free cottage cheese, ¼ c. pepperoncini, 2 tbsp. fresh parsley, 1 tsp. lemon zest and ¼ t. garlic powder pulse or whisk until chunky.

Easy to Make Creole Mayonnaise

Stir 1 tbsp. Creole or Cajun seasoning* into 1 c. of fat-free mayonnaise or Olive Oil Mayo

*Make your own Creole/Cajun seasoning with NO SALT!

Creole/Cajun Seasoning: ¼ tsp. each: cayenne pepper, ground black pepper, paprika, garlic powder or 2 cloves minced or pressed garlic. EASY – YEAH?

Cynthia Bland

Italian Tomato Sauce for Pizza or Spaghetti

This recipe uses no meat. If you can only enjoy foods with meat, do yourself a favor and get ground chicken or turkey. Brown it then use as much paper toweling that is necessary to absorb the fat.

Ingredients

1. Tomato paste
2. Tomato sauce
3. Olive oil
4. Mushrooms (optional)
5. Garlic
6. Onion
7. Italian seasoning (basil, thyme, oregano, fennil)
8. Honey (optional)
9. Red or black pepper (optional)

1. In large sauce pot on high heat put: 1 large can tomato sauce + 1 can water, 1 small can of tomato paste. Stir until smooth. Bring to a boil then reduce heat to low.

Making Eating Right Easy

2. In separate pan put: 2 tbsp. olive oil. When oil gets warm add: 1 large diced onion, 2 cloves diced or pressed garlic, 6 large sliced or diced mushrooms. Saute until onion is translucent (sorta see-through).
3. Add to onion mixture, 1 tsp. thyme, 1 tbsp. parsley, ground or flaked red pepper to taste, 1 teaspoon basil, 1 tablespoon crushed oregano leaves or t tsp. ground oregano. Stir in and sauté until flavors burst (about 5 minutes).
4. Add onion and spice mixture to tomato sauce mixture. Stir in and let reduce for 1 ½ hour on low heat. Stir often. I added a bit of honey to get rid of the tinny taste.

Servings 8.   Calories 108   Total fat 4 gm (sat fat 0 gm); Cholesterol 0 mg; Sodium 34 mg; Potassium 347 mg; Total carbs 17 gm; Fiber 2 gm; sugar 10 gm; Protein 3 gm.

Cynthia Bland

Hot Sauce

Ingredients
1. 5 oz. or about 6 jalapenos, sliced, or your favorite pepper or blend of peppers
2. 1 tbsp. pressed garlic or minced
3. ½ c. diced onion
4. ½ tsp. Olive Oil
5. 1 c. water
6. ½ c. distilled white vinegar

1. Put all ingredients, except vinegar and water, in saucepan over high heat – Sauté for 2 minutes
2. Add water and cook until peppers are soft and water is evaporated. About 20 minutes
3. Pour mixture into blender or food processor and puree until smooth.
4. While mixture is still in blender, drizzle vinegar into it.
5. Strain thru mesh or tea strainer.
   IMPORTANT!
   Pour sauce into STERILIZED JAR with tight lid. Refrigerate at least 2 weeks before using. No preservatives, shelf life is up to 6 months.

Making Eating Right Easy

Healthy snacks

Make your own snacks for 1/8 the price you pay in grocery stores, fast food restaurants and convenient stores (gas stations). You have seen those wonderful yogurt, fruit and granola cups that you buy. Great health benefit. Ridiculous price!

- ➢ Buy a large container of fat-free yogurt, stir into it a little stevia (grow your own to avoid processing chemicals). Splenda (I don't recommend, but it is supposed to be the least toxic of all artificial sweeteners) or ¼ cup of honey and 3 teaspoons of vanilla. You can also put nutmeg or your favorite "dessert" spices in the yogurt or use pureed fresh fruit to create your favorite taste. Layer the granola, yogurt, fruit, granola. You'll have the same food product and enough for several breakfasts. Recipe for granola follows in recipe section.
- ➢ 3 graham crackers with regular peanut butter. 2 tbsp. is a full day's allotment of peanut butter so I use one tablespoon at my first snack time and the second later. The combination of protein and carbs helps stabilize blood sugar.
- ➢ Instead of popping a bonbon into your mouth, pop a few (8 – 9) grapes (red are best for brain function) or 4 – 5 cherries.

- For a "salty snack" use air popped popcorn with "good, healthy" margarine.
- 4 -6 unsalted tops crackers with tad of peanut butter or 1 oz. of low fat cheese.
- Medium potato with fat-free sour cream, low-fat cheese and chopped green onions and pepper – no salt! The cheese and sour cream have a bit.
- 1 serving of your favorite fruit (no bananas unless advised by your doctor to eat them). Medium apple and a serving of melon, approximately twenty diced, not chunks, pieces.
- 1 slice 100% whole wheat bread with 1 tablespoon peanut butter and sugar-free jam or preserves – since sugar –free means an artificial sugar added to the product, use your home-grown Stevia or honey instead of prepared jam/preserves.
- Chopped fruit in your "home-made" yogurt parfait.
- Mix your favorite dried fruits with coarsely chopped walnuts, almonds and pecans. Eat one handful when dying for something sweet or to raise low blood sugar. Still use the bread and peanut butter if blood glucose is really low.
- Your homemade *domuffs*, banana nut bread and other bread desserts in recipe section – watch your serving sizes! These products have carbohydrates!

Making Eating Right Easy
Delicious and Healthy Desserts

You know how you just want a sweet treat sometimes? Well, I've created some muffins that are sweet, tasty and healthy! They taste nothing like the "muffins" that you get in fast food restaurants, at Sam's or bakeries. They are not sugary. You can switch up on the fruits that you want to use. All of them will work just fine. Some fresh fruits have to be steamed before using if you want them cooked soft.

Home-grown Stevia

Not only is it cheaper to grow your own sweetener, there is no "ose" in it. All sweeteners that end in "ose" have sugar: fructose (sugar from fruit and vegetables); lactose (milk sugar); sucrose (cane or beet sugar) dextrose (sugar from starches). Your sweetener has no preservatives or additives. It is pure and natural; the healthiest sweetener you can ingest. No risks.

Go to Walmart's or Lowe's Garden center and purchase 2 Stevia plants.

Transplant them in a pot filled with regular potting soil. Put the pot in full sun. Keep soil damp.

You can begin harvesting the leaves when the plant is about 6" tall. Cut the stems from the bottom of the plant. Remove the leaves and place in shallow bowl in direct sunlight and let dry for at least 12 hours. When leave crumble at your touch they are ready to be processed.

Puree the leaves until they become powder. I didn't process a lot, so I pulverized my dry product on foil with the handle of a knife You can make a liquid sweetener by boiling 3 tsp. of powder in 1 cup of water. Or you can simply put powder directly into your food product. 3 teaspoons of the powder equals 1 cup of granulated sugar, so don't add too much to your coffee, tea or lemonade.

Granola

Great in yogurt for breakfast or snacks. To me, it's much better than cooked oatmeal.

Ingredients
    1. Oatmeal
    2. Milled flax seed

Making Eating Right Easy

3. Honey
4. Olive oil or "good margarine"
5. Nuts - optional
6. Raisins - optional

Preheat oven to 325°

1) Whisk to blend 1/3 cup honey and 2 tbsp. good margarine.
2) In large bowl put 4 cups oats, 1 c. chopped pecans and/or walnuts and ½ c. milled flax seed.
3) Pour honey mixture over oats, nuts, flaxseed and toss to coat.
4) In rimmed pan spread out and bake 30 minutes.
5) Add dried berries, cherries and other fruits.

Serves 28. Calories 131; Total fat 6 gm (sat fat 0 gm); Cholesterol 0 mg; Sodium 1 mg; Potassium 77 mg; Total Carbs 19 gm; Fiber 3 gm; Sugar 8 gm; Protein 3 gm.

Basic Muffin Recipe

Use this recipe and go wild with your favorite "tastes": cinnamon, nutmeg, vanilla, almond flavoring, cocoa, nuts, dried fruit. Do your calculations after you finish having fun. Go to Google and type in *carbs in (your favorite "taste")*.

Cynthia Bland

Ingredients

1. Whole wheat flour
2. Milled flax seed
3. Oatmeal
4. Can of unsweetened applesauce or homemade applesauce
5. 1% milk or fat-free evaporated milk
6. Baking powder
7. Baking soda
8. *Your favorite sweetener,* hopefully home grown and produced Stevia

Preheat oven to 325 degrees

1. Put in bowl #1: 1 c. whole wheat flour, 1c. milled flax seed, 1 c. oatmeal, 3 teaspoons baking powder, 1-1/2 t. baking soda ... Mix until blended.
2. Whisk in bowl #2: 1-1/2 c. applesauce. 1 cup of 1% milk or fat-free evaporated milk, and ¼ c. honey.
3. Stir liquid mixture into dry mixture until well blended.
4. If batter is too stiff, mix in milk choice ½ cup at-a-time.
5. Fill oiled medium sized muffin tins ¾ full.
6. Bake for 40 minutes or until muffin spring back when pressed in the center.

Serves 16. Calories 134; Total fat 6 gm (Sat fat 0); Cholesterol 1 mg; sodium 13 mg; Potassium 00 mg; Total Carbs 19 gm; Fiber 6 gm; Sugars 6 gm; Protein 6 gm

Muffins made with Almond Flour - gluten free

I've used both kinds of flour and gotten the same result.

Ingredients

1. Almond Flour
2. Milled flax seed
3. Banana
4. Egg whites
5. Sour cream or coconut milk
6. Nuts of your choice
7. Olive or coconut oil
8. Baking powder
9. Sweetener of your choice or honey

Preheat oven to 325°

1. Combine 2 cups almond flour (or whole wheat flour), ¼ cup ground flax seed, 1 tsp. baking powder and sweetener.

2. Mash 1 ripe banana until smooth. Whisk in 2 large egg whites beat, ½ cup fat free sour cream or coconut milk, ¼ cup chopped walnuts, coconut oil, or olive oil.
3. Add banana mixture to dry ingredients and mix thoroughly.
4. Fold in fruits of your choice.
5. Bake about 45 minutes. To test for "doneness", insert a toothpick in the center of one. If the toothpick comes out dry, they're ready; but remember, if you use pulpy fruits the toothpick will not come out dry.

Serves 12.   Calories 178; Total fat 14 gm (sat fat 2 gm); Cholesterol 32 mg; Sodium 17 mg; Potassium 63 mg; Total carbs 6 gm; Fiber 3 gm; Sugar 3 gm; Protein 6 gm.

Butternut Squash Muffins

Really good! I just made some. Yum, Yum! You can make these muffins with sweet potatoes using the same recipe. Even zucchini!

Ingredients

      1. Small butternut squash

      2. Whole wheat flour or almond flour

      3. Honey

Making Eating Right Easy

4. Baking powder
5. Nutmeg
6. Cinnamon
7. Milk
8. Eggs
9. Olive oil or "good margarine"

Preheat oven to 400°

1. Peel and dice 1 pound of butternut squash. I used the tubular part (no seeds to remove).
2. Put the diced squash into boiling water and boil for 20 minutes until tender.
3. Drain and puree.
4. Pour into a bowl and whisk in ½ cup honey.
5. In a large bowl, whisk 1-1/2 cup whole wheat flour, 2 tsp. baking powder, 1 teaspoon nutmeg and 1 tsp. cinnamon.
6. Put in medium bowl ¾ cup milk, an egg beaten, and 1 tbsp. melted good margarine, then fold in squash mixture.
7. Fold squash mixture into flour mixture until moistened.
8. Fill tins ½ full. Bake 20 minutes. When they spring back when pressed, they are ready. Center may be moist – squash is a fruit!
9. Google "recipes for butternut squash" to get recipes for the leftover squash.

Serves 24. Calories 65; Total fat 1 gm (sat fat 0); Cholesterol 0 mg; Sodium 7 mg; Potassium 111 mg; Total Carbs 13 gm; Fiber 2 gm; Sugar 4 gm; Protein 2 gm.

Raisin Walnut Muffins

This muffin recipe is very basic. I made these muffins with ¾ c. flaked coconut. The coconut did not change the texture one bit. It just added a little bit of sweetening.

Ingredients

1. Whole wheat flour
2. Oatmeal
3. Milled flax seed
4. Canola oil
5. Fat-free evaporated milk
6. Applesauce
7. Cinnamon
8. nutmeg
9. Baking soda
10. Baking powder
11. Nut of choice
12. Raisins

Making Eating Right Easy

Preheat oven to 325°

1. In a large bowl put 1 c. flour, 1 c. oatmeal, ¼ cup milled flax seed , 2 tbsp. cinnamon, (coconut if you like), ½ tsp. baking soda, 2 tsp. baking powder, and ¼ t. nutmeg. Set aside.
2. In a smaller bowl put ¾ cup applesauce, 1 cup fat free evaporated milk and ¾ cup canola oil. Whisk into this mixture ¼ c. honey.
3. Pour liquid mixture into dry mixture, whisking to blend.
4. Stir in 1 c. chopped walnuts and ¾ cup raisins.
5. Bake until toothpick inserted in middle comes out with no batter.
6. Note: I added ¼ c cocoa to satisfy my taste for chocolate. Good!

Serves 16.   Calories 102; Total Fat 3 gm (sat fat 0 gm); Cholesterol 0 mg; Sodium 18 mg; Potassium 93 mg; Total Carbs 17 gm; Fiber 2 gm; Sugar 7 gm; Protein 3 gm

Coconut Bars

Use this basic recipe without coconut. Substitute the honey with 1/3 cup of molasses to make a tasty, sweet treat. I eat two to three of these nuggets when my blood sugar is low or for a dessert when my blood sugar is no higher than 120.

Ingredients
1. Whole wheat flour
2. Milled flax seed
3. Applesauce
4. Honey
5. Baking soda
6. Baking powder
7. Cinnamon
8. Nutmeg
9. Vanilla
10. Raisins

Preheat oven to 350°

1. In large bowl mix: 2 cups flaked coconut, 1 c. chopped almonds, ½ c. milled flax seed, 1- ½ c. whole wheat flour, ½ tsp. baking soda, 2 tsp. baking powder, ¼ t. nutmeg, 1 tbsp. cinnamon. Add ½ cup raisins for sweetening.
2. In smaller bowl mix ¾ cup applesauce (no sugar added), 1/3 cup honey, 1 tsp. vanilla and ¼ cup canola oil.
3. Pour liquid mixture into dry mixture and knead into ball.
4. Place by teaspoon on cookie sheet, press each cookie with a fork dampened with water.

5. Bake for 7 – 10 minutes for soft nutritious cookie.

Serves 25   Calories 112; Total fat 6 gm (sat fat 1 gm); Cholesterol 0 mg; Sodium 18 mg; Potassium 88 mg; Total carbs 14 mg; Fiber 2 gm; Sugar 5 gm; Protein 2 gm.

Bread Pudding

An Old Time Favorite Dessert served hot with one of two toppings that follow. What makes this dessert so healthy is that it is made with "leftover bread": the ends that most don't want to eat, bagels, English muffins, raisin bread … any kinds of "leftover bread!" So save the bread that you usually give to the birds. I put it in freezer bags and save it until I have the equivalency of 8 slices of bread.

Ingredients

       1. Bread

       2. Fat-free evaporated milk

       3. Raisins

       4. Honey

       5. Vanilla

       6. Nutmeg

       7. Cinnamon

       8. Nuts

Cynthia Bland

Preheat oven to 325°

1. Lay the bread out in the air for a while to remove some of the moisture.
2. When bread is dried out, break it into ½" pieces and put it into a baking pan. In sauce pot put: 1 can fat free evaporated milk, 1 can water, 3/4 cup raisins, 1 cup chopped nuts (optional), 1 tbsp. of cinnamon, 1 tsp. nutmeg, 1/4 cup of honey, 1 tsp. vanilla. Place on medium heat until hot, not boiling.
3. Stir milk mixture and then pour over bread pieces, lifting gently with large fork or spoon until all of the bread is wet.
4. Let pudding sit on top of stove for 20 minutes then put into oven and bake until golden brown (about 1 hour).
5. Serve hot or cold plain or with topping of your choice.

Serves 8. Calories 277; Total fat 10 gm (sat fat 1 gm) Cholesterol 0 mg; Sodium 202 mg; Potassium 434 mg; Total Carbs 40 mg; Fiber 3 gm; Sugar 28 gm; Protein 8 gm.

I eat these plain, but if you like, using lemon sauce or cinnamon sauce add value.

Making Eating Right Easy

Lemon Sauce

Ingredients

    1. Corn starch

    2. Honey

    3. Sweetener of your choice

    4. Lemon

1. In a small sauce pot, Mix 2 tbsp. of corn starch into cold water until dissolved. In a small measuring cup, mix ¼ cup honey, 2 tbsp. of Stevia or Splenda, 3 tbsp. lemon juice and 1 tsp. lemon zest. Stir until blended.
2. Pour honey/lemon mixture into corn starch water and cook on medium heat until sauce thickens.
3. You can substitute lime for the lemon. You can also use 2 tbsp. cinnamon and 1 tsp. nutmeg instead of the citrus fruit for a sauce that is great on any dessert.

Serves 8 (2 tbsp.). Calories 42; Total fat 0 gm; Cholesterol 0 mg; Sodium 1 mg; Potassium 15 mg; Total carbs 11 gm.

Banana-Oatmeal cookies

Ingredients

    1. Oatmeal (You can purchase gluten-free oatmeal)

2. Milled flax seed
3. Bananas
4. Olive oil
5. Vanilla
6. Baking powder
7. Baking soda
8. Cinnamon
9. Nutmeg
10. Nuts

Preheat oven to 375°

1. In bowl # 1 mix thoroughly 2 ripe bananas mashed until smooth, 1/3 c. olive oil, 1 tbsp. vanilla.
2. In bowl # 2 whisk 2 c. oatmeal, ½ t. baking powder, ½ t. baking soda, ½ t. each – cinnamon and nutmeg. ¼ c. milled flax seed.
3. Blend dry mixture into wet mixture. Add finely chopped nuts (I use walnuts and pecans since they are most beneficial. You can also add dried fruit of your choice).
4. Bake until golden brown around edges.

Serves 20 (2 tbsp. dough per cookie). Calories 52; Total fat 4 gm (sat fat 0 gm); Cholesterol 0 mg; Sodium 6 mg; Potassium 68 mg; Total carbs 4 gm; Fiber 1 gm; Sugar 2 gm; Protein 1 gm.

Making Eating Right Easy

Old Fashioned Rice Pudding

Another healthy and delicious dessert that can be served hot or cold.

Ingredients
1. Brown rice
2. Fat-free evaporated milk
3. Raisins or dates
4. Honey
5. Nutmeg
6. Cinnamon
7. vanilla

Preheat oven to 325°
1. Put 2 cups of cooked brown rice in baking dish.
2. In small bowl pour 1- ½ cup of fat free evaporated milk with: ½ cup raisins or diced dates, 1/8 c. honey, ¼ tsp. nutmeg, 1 tsp. cinnamon and 1 tsp. vanilla.
3. Stir milk mixture until ingredients are blended then pour and stir into rice.
4. Top with sprinkle of nutmeg, then bake until bubbly.

Serves 8. Calories 155; Total fat 0 gm; Cholesterol 0 mg; Sodium 56 mg; Potassium 284 mg; Total carbs 33 gm; Fiber 1 gm; Sugar 19 gm; Protein 5 gm.

Strawberry-Buttermilk Domuffs

I don't have the donut baking tins, so I used muffin tins, hence the name "Domuffs." They taste like fluffy cake donuts, just without the hole.

Ingredients

1. Whole wheat flour
2. Milled flax seed
3. Strawberries
4. Sweetener of your choice
5. Canola oil
6. Buttermilk
7. Eggs
8. Vinegar
9. Molasses
10. Honey
11. Vanilla
12. Nutmeg

Making Eating Right Easy

Preheat oven to 375°

1. Combine in Bowl # 1: 2 c. whole wheat flour, 1 tsp. baking soda, ¼ c. flax seed and 1/8 c. Splenda or Stevia. I have 2 Stevia plants growing in my kitchen window. They are thriving! I pick the leaves and mince or put in my garlic press. You get the juice and crushed leaves. Scrape out what is left and put that in your flour mixture. Stevia is 300 – 500 x as sweet as sugar, so you do not need a lot. It is great!
2. Combine with whisk in bowl #2: ½ cup honey, 3 tbsp. molasses, 1 c. canola oil, ¾ c. buttermilk, 1 tsp. vanilla and ½ t. nutmeg, and 2 large eggs whites beaten a bit. Remember the yolk is cholesterol! Better "waste" in the drain, than in your arteries as plaque causing narrowing of your arteries.
3. Add bowl # 2 to bowl # 1 – whisk until smooth then add 1 tbsp. vinegar then mix thoroughly.
4. Fold in ¾ c finely chopped strawberries.
5. Lightly oil donut pan or muffin tins. Fill ¾ full and bake.
6. Glaze while hot with: 1/8 c. honey + ¼ c Splenda, and ¼ cup crushed strawberries stirred until smooth enough to spread.

Serves 18. Calories 204; Total fat 13 gm (sat fat 1gm); Cholesterol 1 mg; Sodium 22 mg; Potassium 181 mg; Total carbs 21 gm; Fiber 2 gm; Sugar 9 gm; Protein 3 gm.

That Thing We Love To Eat!

I am going to share with you the one thing that I never thought I'd get to eat again – candy. I used to buy boxed candy. I read the ingredients and decided that the sugar alcohol was so high that buying the natural sugar variety was OK. Well, it was as long as I ate ½ piece of candy and then two hours later, ate the other half. What torture! I finally decided to make my own chocolate candy. Some that I could enjoy without the guilt. I bought a bag of semi-sweet morsels, melted them down and experimented. The result: a good piece of candy that is as good for me as any other dessert. It's much better than any candy that can be purchased, and it takes care of my desire for chocolate candy while having nutritious ingredients. I still can only eat 1 – 2 pieces because each piece contains 5 grams of sugar plus the carbs from the nuts and other ingredients that I added. I would guess at 7 grams total carbs – the minimal grams of fiber.

Use mint flavoring, almond flavoring, hazelnut flavoring or your favorite flavoring Here is my recipe.

Making Eating Right Easy

Chocolate Clusters

Ingredients

1. Bag of semi-sweet dark morsels
2. Olive oil
3. Homemade granola
4. Nuts of choice
5. Raisins

1. Put 1/3 bag of semi-sweet dark morsels in a double boiler (If you don't have one, put ingredients into a very small pot and rest it in a larger pot filled halfway with water. Just the bottom of the top pot has to be on water.) Pour ¼ cup olive oil and 1 teaspoon of vanilla over it. Melt while stirring over low heat.
2. Into the melted chocolate put ¼ c. chopped pecans, walnuts, or almonds and ¼ c. homemade Granola.* Stir until well mixed.
3. Place by teaspoons onto a cookie sheet. Place candy in freezer and let freeze.
4. Repeat process with the second 1/3 bag and add different nuts, raisins, thawed and well-drained blueberries.

*You can be as versatile in the selection of your "fillings" as you choose. Just keep it as healthy as possible.

Cynthia Bland

Truly No Sugar Added Chocolate Clusters

This recipe saved me a lot of stress. I love chocolate and not being able to have more than a bit at a time caused me anguish. I never liked dark chocolate, so I had to work with this to get it palatable for those of us who like creamy milk chocolate which we cannot have! The ONLY sugar in this candy is what you add: raisins, tad of honey and/or your favorite sweetener, nuts, granola – I enjoy it with sweetener only and favorite fillings. Regarding sweetener. Sweeten to your taste. Keep tasting a drop until you are satisfied. Record how much you needed to make it a real satisfying treat.

Ingredients

1. Bar of Baker's Chocolate
2. Olive oil
3. Vanilla
4. Sweetener (optional) or honey
5. Raisins
6. Nuts

Making Eating Right Easy

1. Break chocolate bar in half and put into "double boiler."
2. Pour 3 tbsp. olive oil, 1 t. vanilla, 3 tbsp. sweetener and/or ¼ cup honey on top of chocolate. Stir after chocolate is melted.
3. Add ¼ cup granola, 1/4 cup raisins and ¼ cup of nuts to melted chocolate mix.
4. Place by the teaspoon onto a cookie sheet and place in the freezer.

That's it! I ate 3 morsels with raisins, honey, nuts and granola and got no appreciable rise in my blood sugar.

Makes 80 heaping tsp. pieces. Serving size 2 pieces.

Calories 33; Total fat 2 gm (sat fat 0 gm); Cholesterol 0 mg; Sodium 0 mg; Potassium 4 mg; Total Carbs 3 gm; Fiber 0 gm; Sugars 2 gm; Protein 0 gm.

Chapter 4

Let's Drink and Be Merry!

The last thing and one of the most important things you HAVE to do is break the addiction to carbonated sugary or diet beverages.

Carbonated beverages cause the following ailments: osteoporosis (softening of bones), cellulite, stomach pain, bloating, tooth decay (strips the enamel off teeth), diarrhea and is associated with low mineral density. The better fizzy drink would be mineral water which contains calcium and magnesium which protect bone density.

Water! Water! Water! Drink 64 oz. every day! Make 16 oz. of water your first thing in the morning drink. After the first 16, have your morning meal and beverage. Every two hours after the first 16 oz., drink another. It only takes 4 servings to get your 64 oz. The benefits are enormous. Remember, two-thirds of your body's composition is water! Water not only flushes your major body organs of impurities, it thins the blood, replenishes electrolytes, provides essential minerals, and keeps your eyes and skin clear.

One liquid beverage I'd encourage you to drink daily ... every morning!

8 oz. of water with only 2 tbsp. of cider vinegar. Not a thrill, but the benefits are huge! This beverage helps balance blood sugar! Cleanses mucus from your body and reduces inflammation! Sounds like joint pain relief that is not a chemical. Isn't it great?

Teas are valuable drinks. Green tea, cinnamon tea, mint tea, chamomile and many others have been used for centuries because

Making Eating Right Easy

of their medicinal value. Don't pollute your tea with sugar; use honey for complete benefit.

Juices have to be consumed carefully because of the high amount of fructose (sugar), but they are a much better choice. You can learn to enjoy vegetable juices and smoothies that you make yourself. Try real hard. It takes time but like bad eating habits, bad drinking habits can be overcome.

Chapter 5

Doing What We Love to Hate

A very recent report claims that exercising is as important, if not more important to healthy living. This report caused me to really think about which, healthy eating or exercising, is most important. For people suffering with diabetes and/or hypertension and obesity, I surmised that they are equally important. The rule is that these conditions are resolved with both, exercising and diet.

Diabetes, hypertensive and obese patients are treated as cardiac patients because of the great toll put upon the heart. If blood sugar is too high, the heart has to act as a cooling system. If blood pressure is too high, the heart (a muscle) has to strain itself to get blood out of it at the proper rate. If obesity is a reality, the heart has to work harder as it fights to get oxygen into the blood stream. If you are huffing and puffing while doing relatively light movements, your lungs are being strained which effects your heart function. It only makes sense that an exercise regimen is as important than your eating regimen. Being healthy isn't easy when you start out on your journey, but becomes a cake walk as you practice thinking healthy.

Any doctor will tell you that a twenty minute exercise program is beneficial to your good health. If you begin exercising, you will be encouraged to exercise more because your breathing will become easier, your heart will beat stronger, your blood sugar levels will drop. As your stamina increases so does your faith in yourself. You will begin so see and feel "The New You."

If you are one of those people who can find every excuse under the sun to not exercise – I can't afford it. I'm too tired

Making Eating Right Easy

when I get home from work. I have to tend to the children and household affairs. I just don't have time. Here are easy solutions to exercise while you go through your daily routine.

1. When cooking: bend from the waist to get food that has dropped to the floor or to get pots and pans from low cabinets. Stretch your back and reach when getting food products and dishes out. While standing on your legs doing prep work, roll your shoulders back and pull your stomach in to make your navel touch your spine.
2. When cleaning floors, carpets, windows or dusting: get on your hands and knees and use wide sweeping strokes. You can also get great benefit from this motion by sitting on your butt with your legs stretched out in a "V" shape. This exercise will stretch your spine and muscles, strengthen your joints and lungs.
3. Walk in the house. You can purchase, for a few dollars, a pedometer to wrap around your ankle to measure how many miles you walk in a day. You want to get to two miles a day. You'll be surprised at how close you are to that just from walking from room to room collecting trash, dirty laundry, turning out lights, and monitoring your children's activities.
4. Always park as far from the store's entrance as you can. Get a cart from the parking lot and push it into the store. Walk up and down each aisle, whether you want something from each aisle or not. Bend down to get items from the bottom shelves. Reach up to get items that are on the top shelves.
5. Use stairs instead of elevators or escalators.
6. Commit to taking your children or spouse for a twenty minute walk in the evening. This is a great way to cool down and reduce stress after those grueling days at work

and just being a busy mom. This is also a great way to bond with your children and introduce them to Mother Nature's great bounty. Look at the clouds to see if you can find any shaped like an animal then watch the cloud dissipate into another figure. This is really fun! Do times table recitation counting by twos, threes, etc., practice spelling words. Homework can be fun! Learning can be exciting. Watch your children's scores rise.

Chapter 6

My Alpha ... My Beginning

I can't wait to send this guide to Dr. Shenoy, my endocrinologist, by whom I was encouraged to beat my disease. My alpha was when he walked into the examining room after reading the results of my blood test and exclaimed, "I want to clone you! All of your levels are perfect!" Loving approval, I became more than committed to being med free! I knew it could happen!

If you are diligent in your quest to eat healthily to be healthy, your diabetes will actually go into remission (dormant, but there to return if you do not stay on task). You will also experience pretty consistent normal blood pressure readings.

As you go forward remember that your response to undue stress causes blood sugar and blood pressure to rise.

Make your eating and exercising a family affair! Get your children and spouse on board with you. Invite them into the kitchen for hands-on food preparation. Make it so much fun that they will gladly learn and understand nutrition and what healthy food choices look like. They will love their lean bodies, clear skin, shiny, strong hair and healthy nails.

If you are diligent in your food choices and preparation and keeping your exercise regimen, perhaps your family members will not have to ever receive the diagnosis of diabetes and/or hypertension nor experience the pain of being obese.

At this last editing, I AM MED FREE! My A1C stays at 6 or below and my weight is consistently at 123.6. My waistline is 30" (less than half the inches of my height of 66"). And I have loads of energy.

Chapter 7

Learn it! Think it! Live it! Success is Around the Corner

I thank God for His guidance as I continue to seek His face and come under obedience. Again, "We have not because we ask not." (James 4:2-3) Ask! Pray! Believe! Know that God only wants what is good for you! Our physical presence is proof positive that we walk with Christ. We will walk with our heads up, shoulders back and the light of the Holy Spirit shining forth to encourage others to take up the full armor and win the battles before them.

I began praying Philippians 4:6-7 about 6 years ago and it has created, within me, a miraculous change. Whenever I find myself engaged in a battle, especially one that I did not start, I pray for peace, joy and harmony, while giving my stressful situation to God. Now, I must confess that I did start the battles of diabetes and hypertension. For years I picked the fight! For years I ate what I wanted; I ate a killer diet: candy, pop, BBQ ribs, all kinds of sausage, potato chips and alcoholic beverages. And that is why I am faced with the giant of disease. This is a lifelong battle.

The scripture Philipians 4: 6-7: Be anxious (worry) for nothing, but in everything by prayer and supplication with thanksgiving let your requests be made known to God. And the peace of God, which surpasses all understanding, shall guard your heart and mind in Christ Jesus. This scripture brings my stress level to an immediate low. And a good portion of peace, joy and harmony.

Be strong and compassionate as you confront those who oppose your quest and share with loving kindness with those who support you as you journey towards the achievement of your quest for good health.

Just last Sunday (September 14, 2014) after praying Philippians 4:6 -7, the day before, God did indeed, give to me the answer to my request. My pastor, Reverend Corey King, Sr., delivered a sermon that put the icing on the cake of taking on stress. He did a sermon based on 1 Samuel Chapter 17 – the story of how a young, small shepherd took down a giant. Yes, David with confidence in God's covenant, a prayerful spirit and 5 smooth stones slew a giant.

God, through this sermon, responded to my request to be motivated to finish this book, to be confident that it is a much needed work, and that He'd guide my mind and heart to express his will of health for all of us.

I offer to you the highlights of the sermon so that you can apply these wise truths in your battle against the demons that visit you to kill, steal and destroy. This is a huge stress reducer.

How I Got the Job
- Pastor: We live in a survival mode: I just want to make it.
- Me: We have not because we ask not. James 4:3 Make your request known to God, in His will.
- Pastor: Be careful to whom you talk before you go to war. If you talk to the wrong person, you will find yourself having to fight that person and the "enemy" (that person with whom you have original conflict). You don't need "back up" when God is on your side. Not one Israelite offered to help David. They were more than willing to offer David as a sacrificial lamb. They were ready to give up and die.
- Pastor: Avoidance doesn't win wars, fights, or disputes.

- Me: Pray for guidance and then confront the issue head on with God's response to your prayers. If your stomach is turning, it's not God! If you have a sense of peace speak gentle words.
- Pastor: Problem won't go away or get better with time.
- Me: Go, resolve the issue with prayer and a full sense of forgiveness – for yourself and the other person.

To win a battle you have to have:
1. A vision of victory. Have incentive to fight. What do you want to get out of the fight?
   Me: Remember it has to be in God's will. I prayed for peace, joy and harmony to free my mind so that I could finish this book.
2. A memory of motivation. How have you defeated challenges in the past? Celebrate the small victories. How you made it through.
3. To remember that the same God that brought you out before will bring you out again.

As you go through this transformation from the oppression of illness to the freedom of good health, try to focus on this scripture and the sermon notes. Go forward in peace, joy and harmony. You will be the victor over disease! You will get where I am.

Epilogue

As you go through this transformation from the oppression of illness to the freedom of good health, try to focus on this scripture and the sermon notes. Go forward in peace, joy and harmony. You will be the victor over disease! You will get where I am.

I am so used to no sugar, fat and salt that I don't miss them at all – I broke my addiction to all! You can too. Take time, take it one day at a time, and learn to enjoy the freshness of the foods that you put in your mouth. Freshness and natural food products make a real difference in the palatability of your foods.

PRAYER, DIET AND EXERCISE ARE THE KEYS TO CONTROLLING DIABETES AND HIGH BLOOD PRESSURE!

God bless you as you go forward seeking His face and a healthy long life.

Now that I've shared all of my secrets with you. ☺ Use them to provide for yourself a new healthy diet. If you don't like the word diet, use menu of delight. Whatever makes you committed to living a healthier life style and achieve and/or maintain a healthy weight.

Because I realize that there is always room for improvement I continue to work on new ideas and methods to prepare food products that I can use in my kitchen to prepare tasty meals and snacks. I'm heading to the kitchen to make the oatmeal cookies! Just the idea of experimenting as I write out the recipe makes me happy. I'm also making all of the dips to take with me to a family gathering in Lawrenceville to share with those I love. We always have chips and store-bought dips! Tomorrow we'll learn to enjoy "healthy junk food" (what an oxymoron) and walk away feeling "light," therefore less guilty.☺

God bless you as you go forward knowing that it is not so hard to be healthy.

Works Cited

American Diabetes Association. American Diabetes Association, 2015. Web. 26 Feb. 2015.

"ChooseMyPlate.gov." *ChooseMyPlate.gov.* United States Department of Agriculture, 02 June 2011. Web. 25 May 2015.

"Diabetes." - *Mayo Clinic.* Mayo Foundation for Medical Education and Research., n.d. Web. Feb. 2015.

"Diabetes Statistics." *PsycEXTRA Dataset* (2011): n. pag. Center for Disease Control, 2014. Web. Feb. 2015.

"Diseases and Conditions." *Mayo Clinic.* Mayo Foundation for Medical Education and Research., 2015. Web. Feb. 2015.

"An Evidence-Based Approach." *RSS 20.* Authority Nutrition, 2015. Web. Feb. 2015.

Goldschmidt, Vivian, MA. "12 Dangerous And Hidden Food Ingredients In Seemingly Healthy Foods." *12 Dangerous And Hidden Food Ingredients In Seemingly*

Healthy Foods. Save Institute, 2015. Web. 01 Feb. 2015.

Gustafson, Timi, RD. "Food Label Literacy - Food and Health." *Food and Health with Timi Gustafson RD.* Solstice Publications, 03 May 2009. Web. 25 May 2015.

"HOW TO RECOGNIZE GMOS ON FOOD LABELS." *GMOFreegirl.* StudioPress, 2015. Web. Feb. 2015.

"Nutrition Analysis." *Cal Dining.* Berkeley University of California, n.d. Web. 26 May 2015.

CPSIA information can be obtained at www.ICGtesting.com
Printed in the USA
LVOW01s0734100615
441756LV00002B/3/P